Supporting Postnatal Women into Motherhood

A guide to therapeutic groupwork for health professionals

LYNN BERTRAM
Practice Counsellor
Steyning Health Centre

Radcliffe Publishing
Oxford • New York

Radcliffe Publishing Ltd
18 Marcham Road
Abingdon
Oxon OX14 1AA
United Kingdom

www.radcliffe-oxford.com

Electronic catalogue and worldwide online ordering facility.

British Library Cataloguing in Publication Data

A catalogue record for this book is available from the British Library.

ISBN-13: 978 185775 733 0

Typeset by Pindar NZ (Egan Reid), Auckland, New Zealand
Printed and bound by TJI Digital, Padstow, Cornwall, UK

Contents

About the author — vii

Acknowledgements — viii

Introduction — 1

Part A: Background and preparations for a postnatal group — 7

1 The world of motherhood — 9

2 Maternal health — 18

3 Planning the group — 32

4 Managing the group — 46

Part B: The six-week programme — 63

5 Session 1: Expectations and reality — 69

6 Session 2: Roles of motherhood — 90

7 Session 3: Changes in relationships — 105

8 Session 4: Parenting style — 123

9 Session 5: Focus on feelings — 142

10 Session 6: Building self-esteem — 158

Epilogue — 177

Testimonials from women who have attended Stepping Stones — 179

Appendices — 181

Appendix 1A: Expectations and reality — 182

Appendix 1B: Listening — 184

Appendix 2: Roles of motherhood   185

Appendix 3: Changes in relationships   188

Appendix 4: Parenting style   189

Appendix 5A: Focus on feelings   191

Appendix 5B: Feelings exercise   193

Appendix 5C: Difficult feelings exercise   194

Appendix 5D: Example of the difficult feelings exercise   196

Appendix 6: Self-esteem   198

Index   199

About the author

Lynn has worked as a Counsellor at Steyning Health Centre for the past 14 years and chairs the Primary Care Counselling Group for the local area. As a result of her work with individual clients, Lynn was alerted to the challenges of early motherhood and the needs of women at this very vulnerable time.

In 1995, she created and implemented the Stepping Stones programme, which explores the emotional transition to motherhood. Stepping Stones provides a forum for women to discuss their feelings and thoughts around the many changes that occur following the birth and provides vital support at this significant life stage.

Lynn is accredited with the British Association for Counselling and Psychotherapy. She has a private counselling practice, and is a tutor at The Raworth Centre, teaching counselling skills to complementary therapists.

Acknowledgements

I would like to thank the GPs and health visitors at Steyning Health Centre for their imaginative foresight in supporting Stepping Stones from its conception to implementation, and for their continued encouragement for this service.

I have learned a great deal from the women who have attended Stepping Stones, and thank them all for sharing their thoughts and feelings so openly in the groups. This book would not have been written without their enthusiastic participation.

I an indebted to Mary Ashwin for her help during the time of writing – her unstinting support and advice has been invaluable. She has both steadied and inspired me on many occasions – thank you.

I am grateful to Maggie Pettifer, from Radcliffe, who has supported me from the beginning of writing, and who has always been encouraging as well as patient!

My family has always supported me in this process and Ivan Bertram has been invaluable in his advice and help with the mysteries of technology.

Finally, I would like to thank the many colleagues and friends who have believed in Stepping Stones and who have made such valuable contributions and suggestions along the way.

For my daughters – Kerry, Faye and Tessa – who inspire me every day.

Introduction

Visit any community in any country anywhere in the world, and you will see ordinary women carrying out the extraordinary task of bringing up their children. As guardians of the next generation, the mothers of today shape the adults of tomorrow. This first relationship in a child's life provides a base line for all other relationships, and so plays a critical role in the child's future.

A child raised in a loving and caring environment, where he knows he is loved and safe, will face the world with confidence and feel able to deal with life's challenges. However, it is not always an easy task to provide an environment for the child to thrive, physically and emotionally. Working in the National Health Service (NHS) as a counsellor in primary care for the past 14 years, I have encountered many clients who attribute their current problems to some aspect of their upbringing or family history. And yet, to an outsider, their family background is often unremarkable. Indeed, children can be very well cared for physically, but their emotional needs may not have been understood or recognised, leaving them feeling insecure or lacking in confidence.

I believe mothers want to do their best for their babies. By the time of the birth, the majority of mothers are excited to meet the new baby, and may have all kinds of expectations about motherhood. However, the demands of parenthood take many women by surprise, and they may feel emotionally unprepared for the task ahead. The joy of her baby, the worries she might encounter, the exhaustion she will inevitably feel, all make this a time of transition when the mother can feel vulnerable and in need of extra support.

It is a testing time, and a woman may attribute her lack of confidence and expertise to her own personal weaknesses or faults, to the way she was parented herself or to her partner's inadequacies. She may judge herself against other mothers she meets, and find herself lacking. She will also be subject to media images of perfect mothers and babies, looking completely content, and may feel anxious if her feelings are very different.

Support at this crucial life stage can be of great benefit to both mother and baby. The mother is entering a new chapter in her life and is getting to grips with her

new role. The more secure the mother feels in herself, the more she will be able to provide a secure environment for her baby. In simple terms, the happier the mother, the happier the baby.

Supportive groupwork

This book is based on groupwork I have carried out since 1995 with women in the early postnatal period. At that time, GPs and health visitors in the surgery where I work as a counsellor were concerned about the frequency of postnatal depression. It was agreed there was a need to support women at this time to enable them to overcome feelings of isolation and anxiety that can often accompany the birth of a new baby, and that can be a trigger for postnatal depression. A discussion group seemed to be a good way of providing support and introducing women to others at the same life stage. After consultation with both the surgery and with new mothers, Stepping Stones came into being.

Having the opportunity to talk about feelings within a safe environment has been an empowering experience for many women who have attended Stepping Stones. Many changes happen following the birth of a child, and the period of transition in the early months can be difficult to manage. Attending a group enables a woman to understand her feelings are very normal, and also provides her with the opportunity to build a support network with other mothers.

Development of Stepping Stones

Initially, Stepping Stones was aimed at women who had been diagnosed with post-natal depression or who were thought to be struggling with life in some way after the birth. However, it very soon became clear that, as all women go through a period of transition and change following childbirth, it would be much more inclusive to offer the group to all new mothers. The demand for this group quickly grew, and it has become a well established, local service that women are keen to use. The group is open to all, and many women return with their second and subsequent babies. Several women with three or even four children have attended with each baby, and have gained in different ways each time.

Women self refer, which demonstrates there is a clear need for support for the mother in the early weeks and months after birth. The women are ordinary in that they are looking after their babies well, and have given no cause for special interest or concern from health professionals. Many women attend following recommendations from others.

The conception of this book

Unlike other groups that provide support, advice and information regarding the baby, Stepping Stones focuses on the mother – her thoughts and feelings on her journey into this new role. Listening to women's stories, respecting their views and honouring their feelings are concepts that provide the foundation to these groups.

Over the years, many women have reported that friends have been envious of the support Stepping Stones has provided, and how they too would have benefited from

such a group. Although practices and traditions around pregnancy, childbirth and childrearing differ depending on individual circumstances, the love between mother and baby, and the desire of the mother to do her best for her baby are common themes.

Feedback such as 'It was such a relief to know that other mothers feel the same as I do' has been consistently given since the early days of running these groups. Motherhood is supposed to be such a happy time, and women can be reluctant to disclose any negative thoughts or feelings, even to themselves. To be able to talk openly and honestly about the difficult times, as well as the good times, is empowering and liberating for many women.

My original intention was to support women in the early stages of motherhood, and I hoped the groups would provide opportunities for future friendships. I did not envisage just how cohesive the groups could become after a relatively short time together. The majority of groups have continued to meet, often on a weekly basis, for many years, and have supported each other up to and beyond the child starting school. When additions to the family have meant the group has grown too large to meet in anyone's home, church halls have been hired or the group has met in parks, swimming pools or other activity centres. They have also supported each other through dark times: miscarriage, stillbirth, relationship crises, family bereavements and trauma are challenges that have to be faced and worked through. I believe this ongoing support and care women have given each other has made a significant difference to all those families.

Stepping Stones has supported hundreds of women, helping them confront and deal with their feelings in the postnatal period. They have often been able to use this increased self-awareness and knowledge to deal with the emotional needs of their children, and have been better equipped to cope with the emotional aspects of future life events.

These unexpected and far-reaching outcomes prompted me to use the Stepping Stones material and philosophy to create and write this book. I realised the issues the women brought to the group were relevant to many families, and yet there did not seem to be anywhere else for women to work through or discuss these common themes. I hope this book fills a much-needed gap: 'normalising' difficult feelings makes them less frightening and easier to cope with, empowering women to confidently carry out the all-important task of raising the next generation.

It is my hope that this book will prompt others to develop similar groups so that other women and their families will benefit from this type of support.

Diversity and difference

The experience of motherhood crosses all cultural, social and economic divides, and so these groups have equal appeal to all mothers, enabling bridges to be built across difference. However, the material may need to be adapted to reflect the make-up of individual groups. Issues of social, cultural and economic difference are further addressed on p. 40.

Although the material in the book has been addressed to mothers, fathers caring

for their babies may find the issues relevant to them also. A male perspective could enrich and broaden discussions in groups. *See p. 39* for more detail.

Intended readership

This book offers the opportunity to explore the experience of motherhood at emotional, intellectual and practical levels and would be of interest to:

+ health practitioners working directly with women at this life stage, including health visitors, midwives, GPs, practice nurses, social workers, community psychiatric nurses, counsellors, clinical psychologists, family therapists, professionals from the child and adolescent mental health team
+ professionals who have dealings with other aspects of family life, for example, pre-school or primary schoolteachers
+ government and voluntary organisations that support the family and women's health, for example, Surestart, the National Childbirth Trust, and the National Society for the Prevention of Cruelty to Children (NSPCC)
+ alternative therapists, including homeopaths, aromatherapists, reflexologists, nutritional therapists, and acupuncturists who have an interest in women's health
+ mothers who wish to reflect on their early experiences of motherhood.

Structure of the book

Part A of the book provides the background to the groupwork. Chapter 1 begins by setting the scene with a case study of a woman who has just had her first baby, and contrasts her experience to that of her own mother. Therapeutic influences on parenting are explored through the work of Bowlby, Winnicott, Stern, and more recently, Sue Gerhardt's work on how affection shapes the baby's developing brain. Chapter 2 looks at women's mental and emotional health during pregnancy and the postnatal period, explores postnatal depression, and reflects on why women find it so difficult to seek help at this time. Chapter 3 gives practical suggestions on starting a group, while Chapter 4 considers the skills and techniques required to manage the emotional content of a group.

Part B sets out the programme: Chapter 5 explores expectations and reality, Chapter 6 outlines roles of motherhood, Chapter 7 looks at changes in relationships, Chapter 8 discusses parenting style, Chapter 9 focuses on feelings, and Chapter 10 examines ways to build self-esteem. A outline plan is included for each session, and a group case study demonstrates how a group might develop over the six-session programme. The facilitator's comments on each session provide further insight on managing the group process. Supporting notes provide more information and high-light recurrent themes drawn from groups over a number of years.

The six appendices include the prompt questions and handouts for each session, and could be given to encourage further thought and discussion. For ease, I have referred to the facilitator and participants as female and the baby as male.

Through Stepping Stones I have been able to observe hundreds of families grow and

develop with the birth of a new baby, and have often been moved by the experiences the women have brought to the groups. It has been a privilege for me to share with them the joy, as well as the challenges, of the first few months following the birth. I hope this book will encourage more thought and understanding about the many exciting yet daunting steps women take in the emotional transition to motherhood.

Lynn Bertram
May 2008

Background and preparations for a postnatal group

CHAPTER 1

The world of motherhood

Congratulations and welcome to a new world that will stretch you to the limits, but also bring you much happiness. Not a job; more a vocation, a way of being that will take you on a journey lasting for the rest of your life. There are plenty of opportunities for expansion in the short term, and promotion later on with lots of challenges and surprises along the way. The demands are high though, as you have to be available 24/7, with no time off. The rewards will be rich and plentiful, although sometimes best enjoyed with hindsight!

Congratulations. You have become a mother!!

Every child has grown within the mother's womb, and mother and baby have gone through the physical birth experience together. No wonder this relationship is so significant for both of them, and can arouse such profound emotions. In this chapter we will meet two women – a mother and her daughter, and contrast their experiences of motherhood 30 years apart. I will then briefly explore some of the concepts that have shaped our understanding of how children develop emotionally and, in particular, the importance of the mother–baby relationship.

Women's changing lives

Women's lives have changed significantly in recent years, and the following case studies describe the world of motherhood for two generations of women – Sally, a new mother, and her own mother, Anne. Their approaches to motherhood are influenced by both their own past experiences and the thinking of the times in which they live.

Sally lives with her partner, Tony, and gave birth to her first child, Chloe, three months ago.

I never really wanted children, so I'm rather surprised to find myself loving this new role – well most of the time anyway. How did I get here?

Mum was only 22 when she had me and I was determined I wasn't going to be tied down by children at that age – if ever! I wanted to do something with my life. Mum always encouraged my sister, Louise, and I to work hard at school to be

able to get good jobs. I did chemistry at university and then went into teaching. I was made head of department when I was 29, and celebrated by buying my own flat. I enjoyed work and went travelling in the summer holidays. By then most of my friends were settling down and beginning to have babies, but I still wanted my independence.

Then I met someone and we were together for about a year, but that was a disaster and left me feeling very raw. I'd had some eating problems in my first term at Uni, and they came back and I lost loads of weight yet again.

I decided I had to take control of my life. Nick had really touched a raw nerve, and I eventually I went to therapy to help me get over him. I couldn't understand why the therapist kept asking me about my family – I was there to talk about how awful Nick was and didn't want to talk about my parents. But eventually it made sense. My parents divorced when I was 15, and I was so angry and hurt with dad for leaving not just mum but ME! I'd been a real daddy's girl and really missed him. I hated him for going off like that and starting another family, and wouldn't go to see him. I think I decided at some level I would never let anyone close to me. Anyway to cut a long story short, I did get my head straight and then met Tony, and suddenly I did want to settle down – it all fell into place.

Having a baby seemed the natural thing to do but it just didn't happen. I was 32 when we first started trying and it seemed so unfair that, now I was ready for a baby, my body was letting me down. After about a year I went to the doctor and she arranged for us both to be checked out. We had loads of tests and eventually I was treated for endometriosis, and I conceived within two months.

And here she is – I sometimes look at her and can't quite believe she's mine. Tony is a very hands-on dad and dotes on Chloe. He had nearly a month off when she was born with paternity leave and holiday so we really bonded as a family. I'm still breast-feeding – which surprised mum as she bottle-fed us – but think I might like my body back soon. No one told me it would be so tiring and that I would eat so much. I feel OK about my body, even though I am still heavier than I was pre-pregnancy, but it feels as if it's doing what it was designed for. I'm hoping my eating problems are a thing of the past, and I'm sure it helps that I am feeling so much more secure and happier in myself.

I intend to go back to work at the beginning of next year for three days a week, and Tony is hoping to work compressed hours so he will have one day off a week to look after Chloe. We will then need childcare for only two days, though we are still debating nursery versus childminder.

Sometimes I feel I am in information overload – there is so much advice out there. I've got Steve Biddulph[1] and Gina Ford,[2] but I'm trying to trust my own instincts more and just follow the advice that I feel comfortable with, without becoming a martyr to it.

I feel closer to mum since Chloe arrived and wish she lived nearby, although I have to remember I was the one who moved away. She adores Chloe, although I'm not sure she likes being called 'granny'. I ask her for advice, but it's a bit out of date – she can't understand why I put Chloe on her back to sleep; she was always

told to lay the baby on her front! How times change.

I got in contact with dad when I was pregnant. It seemed important to connect with him again, and we have made peace. I actually find I like my stepmother and half brothers. I have been able to talk to both parents about the divorce and how it affected me, and it's helped me let go of the anger and bitterness. All this has made me more determined to talk and listen to my children.

Occasionally I feel overwhelmed by the responsibilities of motherhood and the endless decisions that have to be made. Life really has changed forever – I am only beginning to realise just how much. I'm worried I'm turning into a 1950s housewife: the other day I found myself tidying up the sitting room and putting on some lippie before Tony got home from work! Some days I feel bored and lonely, and miss my old life, but then Chloe smiles at me and my heart melts.

I have just received an invitation to go to a postnatal support and discussion group. I'm not really a group person, but met another mum, Caro, at clinic and she has just finished a group. She said it was good to meet other mums and talk about how things really are and how you feel. So maybe I'll give it a go, and Chloe could make some new friends too.

Anne's experiences of motherhood were very different to that of her daughter.

I had always wanted children, and was keen to start a family as soon as Joe and I got married. He was my first love and I was so happy when we bought our first home on the new estate on the outskirts of the town where we had both grown up. I left school at 16 after O levels and went on to secretarial college for a year, and then worked as a shorthand typist in a solicitor's office. I liked my job but was very happy to give up work when Sally came along. That's what women did then and, besides, Joe wanted me at home looking after the children.

I loved being at home with the girls – Louise was born a couple of years later – but it was hard work. Sally seems to have such a lovely time with Chloe, with swimming and music groups. I had to walk everywhere, of course, or get the bus, so everything took so much longer. I had my trusty old twin tub, but I remember nappies took ages to dry in winter – that damp washing smell!

I read my Dr Spock,[3] much to my mum's dismay. We'd all been brought up on a strict regime of four-hourly feeds, and she thought I was making a rod for my own back when I fed Sally whenever she was hungry.

Money was tight and, when the girls went to school, I became a tupperware agent and did parties. Joe wasn't too pleased if I was out in the evening, but I saved the extra money for holidays, and we had some wonderful caravan holidays in Cornwall, which the girls still talk about.

Although life was busy, I felt lonely sometimes and decided to go back to work when Louise started at the comprehensive. I contacted my old boss and he was more than happy to have me back. I was a bit upset that Joe was so unenthusiastic, but eventually he agreed and had to get used to helping round the house a bit more.

This was the early 80s, and to be honest I hadn't given too much thought to all the publicity about the women's movement – somehow I didn't think it applied to me and Joe didn't think much of 'those women's libbers' as he called them. But I know I changed when I went back to work. I was quite envious of these young independent women who were training to be solicitors, and was determined that my girls would receive all the encouragement I could give them to do well at school and develop a career.

Over the next few years Joe and I unfortunately grew more apart. On New Year's Day 1987, he told me he was leaving us to live with his secretary who was five months pregnant. I was initially devastated, although not entirely surprised. I had never quite believed the sudden interest in golf, especially in winter.

To be honest, I was so caught up in my own feelings I didn't think too much about how the divorce affected the girls. Sally was very difficult and would see Joe only if she absolutely had to, but she seemed OK most of the time. She went off the rails a bit but got herself off to university, and I thought we had survived pretty well. We had to move, of course, and I then worked full-time to pay for the mortgage. That period of my life is all a bit of a blur. I think I was in survival mode for years.

Sally was always very independent, but I wondered when she was going to find someone to settle down with and Tony is great - such a loving father. I'm glad she and Joe are talking again, but feel very guilty that Sally was having such a difficult time and couldn't talk to me about it. I still don't really understand why, but we are much closer now, and I'm really looking forward to having a close relationship with Chloe. I hope I'll have more time as a grandmother although I'm still busy at work full-time. I remarried in 1990 and then trained as a social worker, which I love. I would never have guessed how my life would turn out when I got married at 20. I wonder what life holds for Chloe . . .

Anne and Sally are women of their time, both wanting to do their best for their children. They are both 'ordinary' in the sense that, although they have undoubtedly had difficulties to overcome, they both come from loving backgrounds. There is no history of abuse or neglect or very unusual circumstances that would mark them out as being very different from other families in their road. Anne married for life, then her life took an unexpected turn when she got divorced, and she had to forge a different path. Sally has also had to find her own way of dealing with the issues resulting from her past. Motherhood prompted her to re-connect with her estranged father, and develop a more honest and intimate relationship with both parents.

Anne and Joe had provided Sally with a secure and loving environment in her early life and Sally always knew she was loved. This was why it was such a blow for her when her father abandoned her, in her eyes, for another family. Nevertheless, that early solid foundation enabled Sally to ultimately confront and resolve these painful issues. We cannot always protect our children from pain and suffering, but we can provide them with some tools to support them in times of need.

Sally gained valuable insight into her inner emotional life, and learnt about her

own needs and strengths. Her self-esteem and sense of self-worth were strengthened, which enabled her to embark on a healthy relationship, based on respect and equality. Sally's inner security will assist her in providing a secure base for her children.

The baby's emotional world

Our understanding of a child's emotional world and development has increased in recent years, and this sections features some of the theorists I have found particularly helpful.

John Bowlby

John Bowlby (1907–90) was a psychiatrist and psychoanalyst who, throughout his working life, did much to change social policy and influence government thinking on the needs of families and children. Gomez states Bowlby: 'had a more direct effect on British society than any psychoanalyst except Freud'.[4]

Bowlby's trilogy on Attachment,[5] Separation[6] and Loss[7] are classic texts that underpin the attachment theory he developed while working alongside James Robertson, Mary Ainsworth and Mary Boston.

Attachment theory

Attachment theory works on the principle that we all have an innate need for relationship, and this need is met initially by the attachment of mother and baby. The quality of this bonding with the mother and later secondary attachment figures will build a 'secure base' from which the child can enjoy life. Bowlby believed that a security of attachment was 'essential for emotional maturation'.[8] The secure child has 'an inner representation of a lovable self and responsive other, with enjoyable interactions alternating with exciting explorations in an interesting world'.[9]

Bowlby's colleague, Mary Ainsworth, noted how one-year-old babies reacted to separation from their mothers. This is the famous 'strange situation' observation. Mother, baby and observer were all together in a playroom. After a short time, the mother left, returning a few minutes later. Ainsworth was able to identify different patterns of behaviour that reflected the mother's behaviour and responsiveness to her baby. She categorised them as follows.

+ The securely attached group were upset by the mothers' disappearance, and demanded and received attention from her on her return. They then continued to play and explore happily.
+ The insecure–avoidant group did not seem particularly upset when she left, and ignored her when she returned. However, they were unable to get on with their play and watched the mother intently on her return.
+ The insecure–ambivalent group was panicked by the mother's absence, and both clung to her and fought her off when she returned. They, too, did not return to play.

A fourth categorisation was added later.

+ The insecure–disorganised group, which was confused and bewildered by the situation.[10]

Building a secure base is therefore extremely important, and William and Martha Sears describe how 'attachment parenting' can work in a book full of very practical suggestions.[11]

Although attachment theory has made a significant contribution to our understanding of child development, Bowlby's opinions on the risks to the child if placed in full-time daycare have made him unpopular in some quarters. Biddulph continues this debate today.[12]

Donald Winnicott

Donald Winnicott (1896–1971) was a paediatrician turned psychoanalyst who was particularly interested in the emotional development of babies, and in the influence of the relationship between mother and baby. Winnicott viewed human beings as being basically healthy, and had great respect for mothers. He believed they should have as little interference as possible from 'experts'. Instead, healthcare professionals should 'foster the mother's belief in herself' and learn from them, rather than the other way round. Winnicott shared his ideas with the general public in a series of broadcasts and public lectures during the 1950s and 1960s, presenting his ideas in simple and accessible language.

Winnicott believed the foundations for mental health could be laid down by providing the baby with positive experiences of 'holding', (physical and emotional) 'handling' and 'object presenting'.[13] The 'good enough' mother will hold and handle her baby with sensitivity and empathy, and will bring the world to him when he is ready. Winnicott's approach advocates a kind of watchful waiting – being attentive and available to the baby, and yet allowing the baby to take the lead and set the pace. The mother attempts to create a delicate balance between protecting her child while not smothering him, creating a safe environment and yet encouraging the child to create and explore his own world. This enables the baby to develop his 'true self', which indicates strong mental health.

However, if the mother is continually unable to provide this safe environment, the baby may develop a 'false self', whereby 'the child adapts to a mismatch between its real needs and how its parents are able to respond'.[14] The adaptation to others' needs may become an automatic defensive reaction, with which the resulting adult has to continually contend.

Concepts associated with Winnicott
Primary maternal preoccupation

In late pregnancy and during the early postnatal months, the mother becomes completely focused on the baby's needs, almost to the exclusion of everything else. This preoccupation lessens as the baby's complete dependence on the mother decreases.

The ordinary devoted mother

Although he was criticised for being sentimental or idealising mothers, this phrase reinforces Winnicott's confidence in mothers.

The good enough mother

This principle releases the mother from striving to be perfect and so reduces anxiety.

The facilitating environment

The baby is enabled to grow and interact with his surroundings at a pace appropriate for his needs.

The nursing couple

This refers to the intimacy of the feeding experience between mother and baby, and does not specifically refer to breast-feeding. Winnicott saw the mother and baby initially as a single entity, and is reputed to have said 'there is no such thing as a baby, there is only a mothering pair'.

The transitional object

This helps the baby manage his anxieties when his mother is absent. The soft toy or blanket comforts the child and 'is the emblem of the child's internal unity with a giving accepting nurturing mother'.[15] It can represent the mother while belonging to the child.

Daniel Stern

In more recent years, psychiatrist Daniel Stern has also written about how the relationship between mother and baby evolves, and how this relationship enables the baby's sense of self to develop.[16]

As well as writing for a clinical audience, Stern has written directly for mothers to increase their understanding of their 'inner landscape'; exploring this role and how the responses to motherhood brings changes. He describes the mother's progress from pregnancy and birth to motherhood, and the emotional adjustments and challenges she will encounter along the way.[17]

Stern also writes about how the baby begins to make sense of his world. Based on his work within his clinical practice and using what is known about child development, he has written Joey's 'autobiography'. Stern describes Joey at six weeks, four-and-a-half months, 12 months, 24 months and four years. He imagines Joey's inner world and describes how he relates to his parents as he grows and acquires new skills.[18]

Sue Gerhardt

Why Love Matters by Sue Gerhardt explains why love is so important for the baby in the early years, and demonstrates how interactions between parents and baby have far-reaching effects on the personality of the growing child.[19] The orbitofrontal cortex area of the brain, part of the pre-frontal cortex, plays a large part in how we

manage our emotional world. This 'social brain' helps us to pick up on the subtle non-verbal clues we receive from others, which enables us to repond with sensitivity and empathy.[20]

Most interestingly, Gerhardt explains that this part of the brain develops almost entirely postnatally, its physiological development dependent on the baby's experience with those around him. She emphasises that the orbitofrontal cortex does not develop automatically, but develops only as a result of human interaction. Gerhardt cites a chilling study of Romanian orphans whose brains had a 'virtual black hole' where the orbitofrontal cortex should have been. These babies had been left in their cots all day with no close contact with adults, and so that part of the brain had just not developed. It seems unlikely that this damage can be repaired later.[21]

The cooing and gurgling games that occur from the earliest days and weeks between mother and baby help this part of the brain to develop, and prepare the baby for future social dialogue. Most mothers naturally engage in frequent periods of play, but this can sometimes be put aside when other tasks seem more pressing. Perhaps if more women realised its vital importance, they would devote more guilt-free time to this activity, which is pleasurable to both mother and child.

Gerhardt also explains the effects of cortisol on our emotional lives. When we are in extreme stress, our bodies react in a myriad of ways: as adults we will be aware of a range of responses both physical and emotional (racing heart, butterflies in stomach, feelings of anger, fear). What we are not aware of is what is happening inside our bodies. Stress triggers a 'cascade of chemical reactions', and one of the end-products is the stress hormone, cortisol. Whereas adults may be able to develop coping strategies to help manage stress, babies are unable to manage stress on their own, and rely on others to calm and soothe them. A hungry baby's cry will quickly reach fever pitch if they are not fed immediately – they are unable to wait. Hunger is life-threatening to them, and they will do all they can to get the attention they need: at this stage it is likely that the baby's cortisol levels are high. If the baby lives in a loving environment, and their needs are met with care and sensitivity, the baby gradually gains confidence that help will come and the cortisol response is less easily triggered. But if the cortisol stress response is triggered repeatedly, brain development is again affected. Gerhardt states 'early care actually shapes the developing nervous system and determines how stress is interpreted and responded to in the future'.

Although the worlds of psychiatry, psychology and psychotherapy have always been attentive to the effects of the past on the present, Gerhardt presents the concrete evidence that neuroscience has given to us in recent years, and translates it into accessible language.

Bowlby, Winnicott, Stern and Gerhardt have underlined the importance of the mother–baby relationship. How we mother our children is of utmost importance, and women today have many pressures with which to contend. Balancing the needs of the baby with the demands of her relationship, family and work means a woman has to become even more proficient at multi-tasking. But we need to remember that how we parent our children today will have implications for how society develops

in the next generation, and every support should be given to women and families at this crucial period.

References

1 Biddulph S. *Raising Babies: should under threes go to nursery?* London: Harper Thorsons; 2006.

2 Ford G. *The Contented Little Baby Book.* New ed. Vermilion; London: Ebury Press; 2006

3 Spock B. *The Common Sense Book of Baby and Child Care.* 7th ed. New York: Pocket; 1998.

4 Gomez L. *An Introduction to Object Relations.* London: Free Association Books; 1997.

5 Bowlby J. *Attachment and Loss. Vol. 1 Attachment.* London: Pimlico; 1969.

6 Bowlby J. *Attachment and Loss. Vol. 2 Separation.* London: Pimlico; 1998.

7 Bowlby J. *Attachment and Loss. Vol. 3 Loss.* London: Penguin Books; 1991.

8 Gomez, op. cit.: 154.

9 Ibid.: 161.

10 Bowlby J. *A Secure Base: clinical applications of attachment theory.* London: Routledge; 1988.

11 Sears W, Sears M. *The Attachment Parenting Guide: a common sense guide to understanding and nurturing your baby.* New York: Little Brown and Company; 2001.

12 Biddulph S., op. cit.

13 Winnicott DW. *Babies and their Mothers.* London: Free Association Books; 1988.

14 Schwartz J. *Cassandra's Daughter: a history of psychoanalysis.* London: Penguin; 1999.

15 Gomez, op. cit.: 93

16 Stern D. *The Interpersonal World of the Infant.* 2nd ed. New York: Karnac; 1985.

17 Stern D, Bruschweiler-Stern N, Freeland A. *The Birth of a Mother.* London: Bloomsbury; 1998.

18 Stern D. *Diary of a Baby.* New York: Basic Books; 1998.

19 Gerhardt S. *Why Love Matters.* Hove and New York: Brunner-Routledge; 2004.

20 Ibid.: 35.

21 Ibid.: 38.

CHAPTER 2

Maternal health

To begin this chapter we will re-visit Sally and her mother, Anne, for accounts of their experiences of birth and the early days afterwards. I will then outline how a woman's health is monitored during pregnancy, focusing particularly on her mental health and well-being. I shall explore causes and effects of postnatal depression (PND), and draw on the work I have carried out with women in the postnatal period to discuss why it can be so difficult to diagnose. This information highlights areas for future study and research. The chapter concludes with an outlining of how groupwork can enable women to negotiate this important life stage and positively manage the inevitable changes a baby brings.

Sally

Having struggled to get pregnant, I loved *being* pregnant. Although I was very sick and tired in the first couple of months, I didn't mind at all as it confirmed I was pregnant. I worked up to three weeks before my due date and then Chloe arrived two weeks early so I had very little time at home before the birth.

We'd just finished decorating the nursery the week end before! I'd been to classes and really hoped for a water birth, or at least a natural birth. But by the time we had reached hospital I was only four centimetres dilated and couldn't cope with the pain. Tony was great, but I was pretty foul to him and begged for pain relief. It was fine after that but Chloe took her time to get here so I was exhausted, and then had to have some stitches, which was almost the worst bit.

I came home the next day and Tony and I just looked at each other and said, 'What do we do with her?' The first few days were a mixture of highs and lows, and the midwife was lovely and really helped me breast-feed. Of course, we had lots of visitors, which was nice but exhausting as well. Mum stayed for a few days when Tony went back to work – and then I was on my own. That was weird and I'm still getting used to it.

I try to get out with the pram every day, but there's so much to do and then, at the end of the day, I wonder what I have been doing as I will have to do it all again

tomorrow! Still, we're getting there. I signed up for swimming and been to a music club for babies, and I've decided I will go to that group – it starts next Wednesday and hopefully I can meet some other mums.

Anne

As I said, I fell pregnant almost straightaway, but I had a few problems, bleeding and so on, so I was quite anxious for the first few months, and in the end left work early. I was ready to leave and, of course, I wasn't going back after the birth. My mother had had all four of us at home and couldn't understand why I was going into hospital. But I had been worried during the pregnancy and felt safer there.

I found the birth hard and it didn't occur to Joe to be there with me – men weren't in those days. He did his pacing in the corridor, like you see in the old films, and I made do with gas and air. As soon as I looked at Sally I fell in love with her. She was so perfect – I still remember her looking up at me very seriously. Joe visited briefly and then went off to celebrate with his mates.

I think I was in hospital for about three or four days. I was shocked that Sally came home the day after she had Chloe. I went home to mums for about two weeks and she looked after me, but I was glad to get home eventually. Joe was working, of course, and Sally and I had to get on with it.

We went to baby clinic every week and I met Maureen there. Her son was a few weeks older than Sally, and we became good friends and helped each other out. I saw my family every week and gradually I got used to my new life. I worry that Sally lives so far away, but she seems to be coping well so far, and Tony is so helpful with Chloe.

These case studies demonstrate different birth experiences, and changes in the role of fathers and in the attitude of women to work.

Healthcare during pregnancy and the postnatal period

Antenatal and postnatal care in the United Kingdom (UK) follows three National Institute of Clinical Excellence (NICE) guidelines:

1 *Antenatal care: routine care for the healthy pregnant woman*, CG6 2003
2 *Routine postnatal care of women and their babies*, CG37 2006
3 *Antenatal and postnatal mental health*, CG45 2007.

The following provides a guide to the provision of care during a normal pregnancy and postnatal period. Regional variations will be affected by local policy, protocols and staffing levels.

Role of GP

+ The GP is first contact for most medical care.
+ Visit GP as soon as pregnancy is indicated.
+ GP will confirm pregnancy and refer the woman to a maternity unit.

Role of midwife

+ Care is led by the midwife in normal pregnancies.
+ At the booking interview the midwife will:
  — gather all relevant health information, including personal details and a family and medical history
  — carry out a risk assessment.
+ All 'low risk' women will be seen by the midwife on a regular basis to monitor the baby's growth and development, and the mother's physical and emotional health and well being.
+ Women deemed 'high risk' (a current medical condition such as diabetes, or women who have had a previous traumatic delivery) are referred to the hospital consultant.
+ Healthy first-time mothers are usually offered 10 antenatal appointments.
+ Second-time mothers are routinely offered fewer.
+ Post-delivery, midwife contact continues for 10 days after the birth, although this can be extended until 28 days.
+ Care is then handed over to the health visitor.

Role of health visitor

All families with a child under five years old have a named health visitor to advise and support the health and well-being of the whole family, but are best known for their work with mothers and babies. They offer:

+ one antenatal visit
+ one postnatal visit between 10 and 14 days
+ one further contact between six and eight weeks
+ a visit at three months.

They often provide:

+ regular baby weighing clinics, which provide further opportunities for the mother to discuss any anxieties, and also to meet other new mothers
+ postnatal groups dealing with topics of interest and concern, e.g. feeding, sleep and weaning. These groups tend to be baby focused, and are a useful way of providing information and support on a practical level for the inexperienced mother.

Personal child health record

+ A portable record (in the form of a book) of the child's health and development accompanies the child to all medical appointments.
+ The record is given by the health visitor at first contact, ideally antenatally.
+ The book includes a list of minimum contacts, incorporating screening checks and immunisation appointments, that are provided for the child.

Maternal mental health

Although pregnancy and the birth are happy events for many women, some feelings of ambivalence and uncertainty are normal. A qualitative study into postnatal depression in 15 centres across Europe, the United States, Japan and Uganda found that, while new mothers recognised a state of morbid unhappiness as a common phenomenon following childbirth, this was not necessarily viewed as an illness. Support from partners and families was deemed to be the best remedy, with talking therapies being the preferred option if professional help was required.[1]

Antenatal depression

Green and Murray suggest that antenatal depression is as much of a problem as postnatal depression, and seems to be just as common and severe as PND.[2]

- Physical symptoms.
- Tiredness.
- Social support.
- Marital relationship.
- Negative feelings about being pregnant.
- Anxieties about health of the foetus.

BOX 2.1 Factors associated with antenatal depression according to Greene and Murray

Some, although not all, antenatal depression continues postnatally. Women who feel depressed during the pregnancy may find it difficult to have their anxieties taken seriously and be told that all will be well after the birth. Raphael-Leff offers the following chart to highlight possible risk indicators which could be identified during pregnancy and worked through.[3]

Conflicted pregnancies
- Unplanned.
- Untimely (too young, old, early, late).
- 'Wrong' mother, father, baby.
- Acute ambivalence.
- Bipolar conflicts of extreme facilitator/regulator (*see* Chapter 5 for more explanation of these terms).
- Psychosomatic discharge.

Emotional sensitisation
- Post-infertility pregnancy (AIH/AID, IVF, GIFT, ovum donation).
- Family history of perinatal complications.
- Borderline disorders.
- Neurotic defences.
- Psychiatric history.

Complicated pregnancies
- Physical condition of the mother (multiple pregnancies, substance and fetal abuse, eating disorders, HIV positive, illness, disability).
- Life events (bereavement, eviction, miscarriages).
- Socio-economic factors (poverty, housing, unemployment).
- Lack of emotional support.

BOX 2.2 Risk indicators during pregnancy (reproduced with permission from Raphael-Leff J. *Pregnancy: the inside story.* London: Karnac; 1993)

Depression after childbirth

Three types of depression, ranging from mild and common to severe and rare, can occur after childbirth.

Baby blues

These occur within the first few days after birth when the mother feels weepy and low. Baby blues are regarded as normal, and dissipate within a couple of days with no medical treatment necessary

Puerperal (or postnatal) psychosis

This is the most serious and severe type of depression, and usually requires admission to a specialist mother and baby unit. It occurs in one or two women per thousand births. Severe depression may be accompanied by delusions, hallucinations, odd behaviour and irrational thoughts. The woman herself may not recognise she is ill, although it may be clear to those around her. Medical attention must be sought as there is a risk of harm to both mother and baby.[4]

Women with a previous history of depression or psychosis are 50 times more likely to suffer from severe mental illness after having a baby. Women currently suffering from mental illness may stop medication as soon as pregnancy is confirmed, which in turn increases risk to themselves. This vulnerable group requires careful monitoring. Any change in mood must be taken very seriously as a rapid deterioration can occur. Dr Margaret Oates expresses her concern about the risk of suicide for this group of women and the need for increased vigilance to identify them:

> The women who had committed suicide were mostly educated professionals aged 30 and over, with a clear history of psychiatric illness. They mostly chose violent methods, making death a certainty.[5]

PND

PND is a mood disorder that affects between 10 and 15% of women following childbirth. PND usually manifests within the first four to six weeks after birth, but can begin some months later. Although the subject of PND is included in the literature about pregnancy and birth, and also discussed at antenatal classes, most women do not want to consider the possibility that it might happen to them, and so may pay

little attention. This may mean they are not alert to the telltale symptoms when they emerge.

Causes of PND
The Royal College of Psychiatrists' Public Education Editorial Board information leaflet lists the following circumstances that may increase risk of PND:
+ previous depression, especially PND
+ a partner who is not supportive
+ a premature or sick baby
+ loss of own mother during childhood
+ experience of several stresses during a short time period, e.g. housing, financial, employment problems or a recent bereavement.

Lyons-Ruth believes the quality of the relationship the woman had with her own mother in childhood is also a most significant factor.[6]

Protection from PND
While it may not be possible to prevent PND, it may be feasible to limit its damage. Helpful factors are:
+ high self-esteem[7]
+ a single close and confiding relationship[8]
+ support from relevant professional colleagues and services, family and friends, local self-help groups, together with early intervention.

Symptoms of PND
+ Low mood.
+ Irritability.
+ Tearfulness.
+ Unable to enjoy anything.
+ No energy.
+ Lack of interest in self and baby.
+ Feelings of isolation.
+ Reduced libido.
+ Exhaustion but may be unable to sleep.
+ Anxiety particularly around the baby or about own health.
+ Feelings of guilt and failure.
+ Unable to cope leading to feelings of inadequacy.
+ Poor concentration.
+ Thoughts of harming baby.
+ Suicidal thoughts.
+ Self-harm.

A mild form of some of these symptoms is common in the early days, making it difficult to identify when normal reactions deteriorate into depression.

Diagnosis and treatment of PND

The Edinburgh Postnatal Depression Scale (EPDS) was designed as a screening tool to aid health professionals identify depression. While not replacing clinical judgement, the EPDS provides an opportunity for the woman to open up about her feelings.[9]

In February 2007, NICE issued guidance on the diagnosis and treatment of mental health problems during pregnancy and in the first year after birth. The guidelines (*Antenatal and postnatal mental health*, CG45) centred on three questions:

> During the past month, have you often been bothered by feeling down, depressed or hopeless?
>
> During the past month, have you often been bothered by having little interest or pleasure in doing things?
>
> If the woman answers yes to either question, a third question should be considered:
>
> Is this something you feel you need or want help with?

These questions should be asked by health professionals at the woman's first contact with primary care at the start of the pregnancy, and postnatally, usually at four to six weeks and at three to four months. This latest NICE guideline acknowledges that the mother's mental health is just as important as her physical health.

NICE does not recommend the EPDS to be used as a screening tool, but suggests it could form part of a mood assessment together with professional judgement and a clinical interview.

Managing PND

The difficulties facing the depressed mother are compounded by the all-consuming demands of the baby, coupled with a disrupted sleep pattern.

Increased support
+ From family and friends.
+ Accepting help with domestic chores and responsibilities.
+ Talking to a trusted confidante about feelings.
+ Health visitors can offer an empathic listening ear and work in partnership with the mother to support and empower her, as well as being a source of practical parenting advice.

Self-help
+ Exercise: a walk with the baby can be good for both.
+ Eating regular and nutritious meals.

Antidepressants if the depression is moderate or severe

✦ It can take two to four weeks before any apparent benefit is gained from antidepressants.
✦ A normal course of treatment is six months (www.patient.co.uk).

Some antidepressants come out in breast milk, which means the mother may have to choose between breast-feeding and drug therapy. Breast-feeding women are often reluctant to take any medication, even if known risks are small.

> The value of breast-feeding is strongly promoted, and usually gives a sense of satisfaction to the mother that she is giving her baby the best possible start in life. For the mother who already feels she is failing (a common symptom of depression), stopping breast-feeding may only add to her distress, and so may not be considered a viable course of action.

Talking therapies

The following may be offered by the GP, depending on local availability.
✦ Counselling.
✦ Cognitive behaviour therapy.
✦ Psychotherapy.

■ Psychological treatments should be offered within one month of assessment and no longer than three moths afterwards.
■ Antidepressants may be offered if the depression is rated as moderate or severe. Comprehensive guidelines are included on the use of psychotropic medication for pregnant and breast-feeding women to enable a decision to be made which balances the risks and benefits

---

BOX 2.3 NICE guidance for GPs

Effects of PND

Depression is a debilitating illness and PND can have far-reaching effects on all aspects of family life.

Relationship with the baby

Sue Gerhardt describes the baby as incomplete at birth.[10] She likens him to a seedling needing the right conditions for healthy growth. The baby will respond to whatever is offered – this becomes his normal. *The Social Baby* by Murray and Andrews illustrates how the relationship between mother and baby develops through play.[11] A series of photographs demonstrates how mother and baby interact during playtime – each is sensitive to the other and contributes to the progress of the game. This social interplay fosters a sense of security in the baby, and promotes trust and therefore emotional growth. The mother's empathy for the baby and the baby's growing trust in the mother during day-to-day care fosters a secure attachment. The growing child

is likely to grow up with confidence and high self-esteem, and is equipped to deal with life stresses while also having the confidence to ask for help when necessary.

However, when communication with the baby is repeatedly mismatched, and his signals are ignored or misinterpreted, the baby becomes confused and may become distressed or withdrawn. This may lead to an insecure attachment, and the growing child may have little confidence in himself to cope with life's difficulties and may struggle with low self-esteem. Feelings may be difficult to manage and he may exaggerate or suppress them. His ability to demonstrate empathy may be limited, which inevitably will have a negative effect on future relationships.

Depression can adversely affect the ability to communicate effectively. Women suffering from symptoms of depression may find it difficult to develop the kind of attentive and sensitive relationship with her baby to foster a secure attachment. Tronick and Weinberg describe two different patterns of interaction between the depressed mother and her baby.[12]

+ The 'intrusive' mother will handle the baby roughly, speak in an angry tone and actively interfere with their babies activities. The babies spend much of their time looking away from the mother and cry infrequently. These infants 'internalise an angry and protective style of coping . . . [and] are easily angered when interacting with their mother'.
+ Withdrawn mothers are unresponsive and disengaged, and do little to support their babies' activities. Their babies are more likely to be distressed and, although initially become angry, this gives way to a more passive and withdrawn way of coping.

In both cases, the babies seem to mimic the mothers' responses, and it seems likely that these ways of interacting may continue and become normal for the child.

Garber and Dodge found that, when depressed people were faced with problems with others, they either withdrew or attacked them aggressively.[13] Another study indicates that by early childhood, children of depressed mothers have a 29% chance of developing an emotional disorder compared to 8% of children with a medically ill mother.[14] So, the baby of a depressed mother will come to expect low levels of stimulation and a lack of positive feelings.

Effects on cognitive development
Hay believes that some children's cognitive development is permanently affected by PND.[15] He defines intelligence as the capacity to learn, and believes any social experiences that interfere with the baby's developing ability to attend to his environment will affect his intellectual abilities and capacity for learning in later childhood. His review of recent studies confirms his worries and highlights that gender seems to play a role in that boys may be more affected than girls.

Effects on relationship with partner
A depressive illness is very self-absorbing, and the sufferer often withdraws into herself, impairing her ability to empathise or see another perspective. Living with a partner

suffering from depression can be wearing, requiring patience and understanding. The partner of a depressed mother will also need to be able to offer practical help in caring for the baby and with domestic chores, as well as emotional support.

New fathers will vary in their abilities to provide this as they themselves get to grips with their new role and responsibilities. They will often also be juggling work commitments with the demands of home life. If the father is able give this level of support, this will provide the baby with a more normal way of interacting that will help counterbalance a depressive way of communication.

Perhaps predictably, Coyne *et al.* found that many spouses of depressed women were found to be depressed themselves, and reported feeling stressed by their partner's lack of interest in social activities, persistent fatigue, feelings of hopelessness and chronic worrying.[16] Interestingly, in the same way that Lyons-Ruth found the relationship with the woman's own mother to be predictive of depression, so Lovestone and Kumar found that the single most significant factor in male postnatal mental illness was the father's relationship with his own father.[17]

Research findings

Research into the effects of PND undoubtedly indicates negative influences on the mother, the child and the family in the short term and also longer term. It is to be hoped that this information can be used to inform future planning and development of services for women during this vulnerable life stage.

But, however useful this information is to policy makers, mothers themselves often react by taking full responsibility and blaming themselves for causing difficulties for their children. Margaret Oates comments on how 'child-bearing women have been subject to proscriptions and prohibitions of their activities', and how guilt is automatically felt by the mother if things go wrong for any reason.[18] Prescriptive guidance may have the intention of allaying anxiety, but can in fact induce and increase it.

Difficulties with diagnosing PND

> More than half the cases of postnatal depression are unrecognised by GPs and Health visitors.[19]

There is undoubted stigma against any kind of mental health problem, and PND seems to carry even more stigma than a diagnosis of depression at other life stages. Although women have regular contact with health professionals who are aware of the need to monitor the woman's emotional health and well-being, PND can still be missed.

It is more likely that women will open up about their feelings if a trusting relationship is established with one person, for instance her health visitor or GP. In some areas, staffing levels may mean the mother sees different members of the primary care team, and so this rapport does not develop.

If the mother says she is coping and appears to be coping, it will often be assumed she **is** coping, putting the onus on her to seek help.

Dr Michelle McCarthy's research into the acceptance and experience of treatment for postnatal depression in Australia discovered that:[20]

+ most women reached crisis point before seeking help
+ some felt they could no longer look after their babies or no longer wanted their babies
+ some had become suicidal, requiring hospitalisation.

She suggests that the characteristics of depression:

+ negative thinking
+ hopelessness
+ lack of self-esteem
+ decreased motivation

make it very difficult for the woman herself to recognise PND and so to actively seek help from health professionals.

Obstacles to seeking help

♦ Parenthood is often anticipated with excitement and high expectations.
♦ Difficulties in conceiving or any previous experiences of miscarriage or stillbirth may increase the expectations and hopes for this child even further.
♦ The mother may be shocked at her feelings of unhappiness and find it difficult to admit to feeling so low when she *should* be feeling so happy. The guilt and shame around these feelings only add to her distress, and prevent her from admitting how she really feels – even to herself
♦ Women used to coping, who see themselves as strong and organised, and who have aspirations to 'be perfect', may find this new state of mind destabilising and expect to be able to 'snap out of it'. If those around her are also used to her being in control, they too may be unsettled by the changes in her.
♦ The father and close family may be delighted with the new baby, making it impossible for the new mother to disclose how she really feels.
♦ If the woman is the emotionally stronger one in the partnership, she may not be able to lean on her partner for support, and may feel she must keep her anxieties to herself.
♦ She may fear criticism from others, and be very worried about being seen as not coping.
♦ She may judge herself harshly as a 'bad mother', and feel lacking in confidence in her mothering skills, which will further lower her self-esteem.
♦ Family or friends may be struggling with fertility issues or even be coming to terms with childlessness, making it impossible for her to 'moan' about her circumstances – she's so lucky to have such a beautiful baby.
♦ If she mixes with other new mothers, she may imagine everyone else is coping well, increasing her sense of inadequacy.
♦ She may ultimately fear losing her baby if she admits to her feelings. This is extremely

unlikely and, while the majority of women know this at an intellectual level, it can present a real fear at an emotional level.

♦ She may not be fully aware of the signs of PND: she may have skipped that chapter in the book or not really taken in the information at the antenatal class.

♦ She may discount her feelings, perhaps associating exhaustion, lack of energy and tearfulness with lack of sleep. She may only realise there is a problem when the baby begins to sleep through and her symptoms do not improve.

Women have also reported that memories of the past arise unbidden at this time. This means she may find herself, quite unexpectedly, struggling with painful emotional issues that colour her abilities to be fully in the present:

♦ a past termination
♦ previous abuse – sexual abuse or assault in particular
♦ issues of loss – especially loss of her own mother.

She may find these memories too overwhelming to confront, and do her best to suppress them and so avoid seeking help.

A time for change

Having a baby brings about a major life change, which can be difficult to fully appreciate or plan for during pregnancy. Change, even exciting and positive change, always involves loss: the joy of becoming a family involves the loss of being a couple, the responsibility of being a mother means always having to think about someone else and the loss of being completely carefree.

The early postnatal months bring many changes and challenges, gains and losses to the new parent, and it is important to recognise rather than ignore the feelings around loss, as well as celebrating the gains. This is a normal transitional process and, if these changes can be explored in a non-threatening way, the feelings can then be acknowledged, worked through and released.

The value of groupwork

> To mother generously, a mother needs to feel mothered.[21]

Motherhood is all about giving. The needs of the baby are all-consuming but it must be recognised the mother needs support to be able to give generously to her baby. While this extra support may be supplied by her partner, family and friends, attending a group can help the mother develop into her new role and fulfil some specific needs.

♦ Social support combats loneliness and isolation. Even if the mother is planning to return to work, there is a likely to be a period at home when she cares for the baby full-time. The need for adult company may be a surprise for some women who see themselves as quite self-sufficient.

✦ Psychological support from other women provides encouragement and validation. Stern views motherhood as a craft and calls this psychological support an 'affirming matrix'.[21] This may be provided by more experienced mothers, or by peers.

✦ Exchanging information and observing other mothers in action builds confidence.

✦ Sharing experiences fosters a sense of belonging and connection.

✦ Listening to each other helps establish a network of support.

The facilitator creates a safe environment for discussion, provides reassurance to the inexperienced mother and gives her space to explore her feelings. Once women realise they are not alone in how they feel, they are more able to relax and let go of some of the pressures they may have imposed on themselves. Women who attend a group and form relationships with other women in the same situation are less vulnerable to PND and more able to enjoy their babies. Groupwork can provide a brief, but significant and nurturing, experience for the emerging mother.

The following two chapters outline the tasks involved in planning a postnatal support group and the skills required to run such a group successfully.

References

1 Oates M *et al*. Postnatal depression across countries and cultures: a qualitative study. *British Journal of Psychiatry*. 2004; **184**: s10–16.

2 Green JM, Murray D. The use of the Edinburgh Postnatal Depression Scale in research to explore the relationship between antenatal and postnatal dysphoria. In: Cox J, Holden J, editors. *Perinatal Psychiatry*. London: Gaskell; 1994: 180–98.

3 Raphael-Leff J. *Pregnancy: the inside story*. London: Karnac; 1993.

4 www.patient.co.uk (accessed 13 July 2007).

5 www.repsych.ac.uk (accessed 13 July 2007).

6 Lyons-Ruth K. Maternal depressive symptoms, disorganised infant–mother attachments and hostile–aggressive behaviour in the preschool environment: a prospective longitudinal view from infancy to age 5. *Rochester Symposium on Developmental Psychopathology*. 1992; **4**: 131–71. Quoted in Gerhardt S. *Why Love Matters*. Hove and New York: Brunner-Routledge; 2004.

7 Hobfoll SE, Lieberman M. Personal relationship, personal attributes and stress resistance: mothers reactions to their child's illness. *American Journal of Community Psychology*. 1988; **16**: 565–89. Quoted in Cox J, Holden J, editors. *Perinatal Psychiatry*. London: Gaskell; 1994: 67.

8 Cohen S, Wills TA. Stress, social support and the buffering hypothesis. *Psychological Bulletin*. 1985; **98**: 310–57. Quoted in Cox J, Holden J, editors. *Perinatal Psychiatry*. London: Gaskell; 1994: 67

9 Cox J, Holden J, editors. *Perinatal Psychiatry: use and misuse of the Edinburgh Postnatal Depression Scale*. London: Gaskell; 1994.

10 Gerhardt S. *Why Love Matters*. Hove and New York: Brunner-Routledge; 2004.

11 Murray L, Andrews L. *The Social Baby*. Surrey: CP Publishing; 2000.

12 Tronick EZ, Weinberg MK. Depressed mothers and infants: failure to form dyadic states of consciousness. In: Murray L, Cooper PJ, editors. *Postpartum Depression and Child Development*. New York: Guildford; 1997: 54–81.

13 Garber J, Dodge K. *The Development of Emotional Regulation and Dysregulation*. Cambridge: Cambridge University Press; 1991. Quoted in Gerhardt S. *Why Love Matters*. Hove and New York: Brunner-Routledge; 2004.

14 Hammen C, Burge D, Burney E, *et al.* Longitudinal study of diagnoses in children with unipolar and bipolar depression affective disorder. *Archives of General Psychiatry.* 1990; **47**: 1112–117. Quoted in Gerhardt S. *Why Love Matters*. Hove and New York: Brunner-Routledge; 2004

15 Hay DF. Postpartum depression and cognitive development. In: Murray L, Cooper PJ, editors. *Postpartum Depression and Child Development*. New York: Guildford; 1997: 85–110.

16 Coyne JC, Kessler RC, Tal M, *et al.* Living with a depressed person. *Journal of Consulting and Clinical Psychology*. 1987; **55**: 347–52. Quoted in Murray L, Cooper PJ, editors. *Postpartum Depression and Child Development*. New York: Guildford; 1997: 154.

17 Lovestone S, Kumar R. Postnatal psychiatric illness: the impact on spouses. *British Journal of Psychiatry*. 1993; **163**: 210–16. Quoted in Raphael-Leff J. *Pregnancy: the inside story*. London: Karnac; 1993.

18 Oates M. Adverse effects of maternal antenatal anxiety on children: causal effects or developmental continuum. *British Journal of Psychiatry*. 2002; **180**: 478–79.

19 The Psychiatry Research Trust www.iop.kcl.ac.uk (accessed 13 July 2007).

20 www.news-medical.net (accessed 13 July 2007).

21 Raphael-Leff J, op cit.

22 Stern D, Bruschweiler-Stern N, Freeland A. *The Birth of a Mother*. London: Bloomsbury; 1998.

CHAPTER 3

Planning the group

This chapter explores the steps necessary to plan a support group suitable for women in the postnatal period. Starting a new group requires careful research and preparation, and may take a considerable amount of time. The chapter concentrates on practical processes that need to be put into place at the outset to provide a robust, external structure for the group.

What type of group?

A psycho-educational group is not a therapy group, not an educational group and not a social group, but a mixture of all three.

A therapy group encourages participants to talk about feelings and provides a safe place to express those feelings. Yalom identifies some of the benefits of group psychotherapy as:[1]

+ installation of hope
+ universality – understanding one is not alone
+ imparting information
+ altruism – experiencing the ability to give as well as receive help and support
+ developing social skills, including learning to express feelings
+ imitative behaviour – how the facilitator behaves will act as a role model
+ challenging old patterns – especially reworking old family patterns
+ building interpersonal relationships
+ developing a sense of belonging.

An educational or learning group is more structured, and usually consists of a teacher–pupil relationship with a prepared lesson plan and specific goals and learning outcomes.

A social group provides the opportunity to meet and get to know other people in a relaxed and friendly atmosphere.

A psycho-educational group combines all these elements, and offers:

+ an opportunity to meet others in the same situation
+ time to talk about experiences and feelings.

As a result women can:
+ learn from the experience of others in the group
+ build confidence in this new role
+ feel empowered by taking responsibility for their own and their family's health.

Getting started
Some initial research may need to be carried out to assess the viability of a group.

Local research
Before planning begins it is important to find out what is already available, and to identify any gaps in current service provision. Information can be sourced from:
+ health professionals, e.g. midwives, health visitors, GPs, counsellors
+ providers of childcare, such as child minders, nursery nurses
+ suppliers of social and educational services, e.g. toddler groups, pre-school groups
+ government bodies and charities supporting families, e.g. Surestart, NSPCC, National Childbirth trust (NCT).

It is also useful to consult directly with potential service users, as they will often generate ideas and suggestions based on their actual needs, rather than what others think they might or should need. While women who are already mothers will be able to make suggestions on what support they could have used, pregnant women can supply ideas on how best the group can be marketed and advertised. Contact can be made via the following classes and activities:
+ antenatal and postnatal classes
+ yoga for pregnancy and the postnatal period
+ exercise classes for antenatal and postnatal care
+ music, swimming, baby massage groups for babies.

Forming good relationships with local health professionals at an early planning stage is valuable, and will be beneficial later when the group is advertised. Occasionally, unforeseen problems can be encountered with health professionals who may feel their 'territory' is being invaded or threatened, and may react defensively or even aggressively. They are much more likely to be interested and supportive if the proposed group is viewed as an additional resource for clients, which may then indirectly reduce their own, all too often heavy, workload.

Gathering information
A questionnaire is a quick, easy and cost-effective way to gain information from a large group of people that can be collated and used for future planning. Questionnaires can be distributed directly to potential client groups or via health professionals. A central box for collection of questionnaires can be used to keep costs low. Consider the following in the design of the questionnaire:
+ tick boxes are easily analysed, but may restrict responses

+ open questions provide the opportunity to answer more freely
+ ensure questions are clear and relevant, covering both past experience, suggestions for improvement and future innovation.

The following questionnaire could be distributed among new mothers to gauge their experience and need. It will highlight areas of need and will gauge the level of interest in a support group.

Sample questionnaire

We are looking into the range of services offered to women in the early postnatal period and would be grateful if you, as a new mum, would complete this questionnaire. We would really like to know your views on what helped you adjust to parenthood, and the information you give can be taken account in planning future support. This questionnaire will highlight areas of need and will gauge the level of interest in a support group.

Please think back to your pregnancy and the first few months of your baby's life, and give as much detail as you can.

1. Who did you turn to for help and advice?
   + Your family
   + Health professionals (e.g. GP, midwife, health visitor)
   + No one
   + Other (please specify)

2. Did you gather information from any of the following?
   + Books
   + Magazines
   + Internet
   + Television programmes
   + Other (please specify)

3. Who did you share your worries and concerns with?
   + Your partner
   + Your family
   + Health professionals (e.g. GP, midwife, health visitor)
   + No one
   + Other (please specify)

4. Where did you meet other new mums?
   + Antenatal class
   + Hospital
   + Baby clinic
   + Postnatal group

- ◆ NCT activities
- ◆ Mother and baby/toddler groups
- ◆ Other (please specify)
- ◆ Have not met any new mums

5. Can you remember how you felt during this time? Where would you place yourself on the following scales?

Happy	Sad
Energetic	Exhausted
Calm	Agitated
Confident	Unsure
Relaxed	Tense
Supported	Isolated

6. What would have helped you during this time?
- ◆ More help and support from family and friends
- ◆ More help and support from health professionals
- ◆ More information
- ◆ Meeting other new mums
- ◆ Support from more experienced mums
- ◆ Other (please specify)

7. Would you have been interested in joining a discussion group to support you in adjusting to all the changes that a new baby brings?
- ◆ Yes, definitely
- ◆ Maybe
- ◆ Not at all

Can you give reasons for your answer?

Thank you for your time. If you are prepared to talk in more detail about your experiences during the postnatal period, please complete your personal details and we will contact you.

Name: . . . .

Telephone number: . . . .

Email address: . . . .

Building the group identity

Once the research confirms the need for the group, more detailed planning can begin. A mission statement will describe the aims and objectives of the group and encapsulate the intentions and ethos of the work. The mission statement is likely to be the first item of any proposal application and so must be interesting enough to encourage the reader to find out more. Choose the following:

+ the name – almost as difficult as choosing a name for a baby! An upbeat optimistic name will invite interest
+ the logo – a simple drawing or symbol will draw attention to advertising material and encourage onlookers to read the wording
+ the explanation – to sum up what the group offers.

The name, logo and explanation should appear on all advertising material, letterheads, business cards, and so on.

Funding

In a climate of scarce resources, successful applications need careful planning and research. All the issues discussed in this chapter are relevant to the funding application, and the more detailed the planning stage, the more likely the application will be to succeed.

A funding application should demonstrate how the service fulfils client needs, and provide evidence to establish cost effectiveness of the service. The proposed group offers a preventative intervention when all too often services are concentrated at the more acute end of the spectrum. Research highlighting the difficulties in diagnosing PND and the long-term effects of PND, emotionally, socially and financially, will give most strength to arguments for this type of service.

Many possible avenues for funding exist:

+ statutory bodies, including health, education and social services
+ local government bodies, such as district councils
+ mental health and children's charities
+ lottery or other sources of charitable funding.

The reference section in the library holds directories of grant-making trusts and UK companies that may be worth approaching.

Each application for funding needs to be individually tailored to match the set criteria. This is a time-consuming process requiring expert skills. Advice on how to make funding applications can be obtained from local voluntary service agencies.

A budget breakdown should include the following:

+ funding the planning stage
+ facilitators' fees to include time for administration and supervision
+ room rental and additional costs, including refreshments
+ advertising
+ stationery and postage.

Charges to the client

To offset some of the expense, a charge may be made directly to the participants. Paying a fee for the service demonstrates a commitment from the participants, but may then exclude or discourage some women from attending. However, a nominal weekly charge towards general running costs is reasonable and need not exclude anyone from attending.

The fee charged will vary depending on the locality, and it may be an idea to keep it in line with other groups, for example, the local toddler group. However, it may be that in some areas some women will be unable to contribute and sensitivity needs to be shown. Asking for a weekly voluntary contribution and providing a box or pot where women can put the money in themselves will ensure no one need feel awkward about non-payment.

Summary of tasks to assess viability of a group.
- Research what is already available.
- Make contact with local health providers in both the statutory and voluntary sectors.
- Gather information from potential service users.
- Create and develop the group identity.
- Explore funding sources.
- Calculate budget breakdown.
- Write proposal for group to gain approval on principle.

BOX 3.1 Tasks for the initial planning stage

More detailed planning

Once a need has been identified and some preliminary commitment made, more detailed planning needs to be conducted.

The target group

- ✦ Women in the early postnatal period.
- ✦ Mother and baby need to be accommodated as most women do not want to be parted from their babies in the very early months.
- ✦ The group provides the growing baby with some social interaction.
- ✦ The facilitator can observe the developing relationship between mother and infant, and offer increased support if appropriate.

Confidentiality

Groups that invite disclosure of personal thoughts and feelings must offer confidentiality to individuals, and this must be considered during the earliest stages of planning. *See* pp. 54–5 for a discussion of the group contract and issues of confidentiality.

Benefits of an 'open to all' policy
+ It is inclusive and gives vital support at a major life transition.
+ Self-referral is empowering.
+ Postnatal depression can be more easily detected, instead of remaining hidden.

Who may not be suitable?
+ Women suffering from PND may find a group too daunting at the acute stage of the illness, but it is important they are given a choice. The group may still be beneficial to them at a later date.
+ Women with severe mental health issues may find a group situation intimidating and may benefit more from one-to-one work.

When to plan the group
+ Avoid holiday periods, e.g. Christmas, August.
+ Plan around local school holidays if possible.

When to attend the group
+ The first few weeks after birth are always busy, but after the first month or so, the new mother may begin to feel rather lonely and isolated, and in need of some adult company. This is a vulnerable time, when PND can develop if these feelings continue without detection or support. An invitation to a group can be a valuable link to the outside world, and provide a focus and the beginning of a structure to an otherwise chaotic week.
+ Consider an upper age limit for babies. At eight to nine months, babies become more mobile and vocal, making a flowing group discussion disjointed.
+ An age range of babies means women can receive and give support to each other. This promotes and builds confidence and self-esteem in individuals, and ensures a sense of bonding as the group progresses.

Mixed groups
+ A group for first-time mothers means that all participants are experiencing the same life change at around the same time.
+ The inclusion of second-time mothers and beyond increases the knowledge base within the group and encourages women to learn from each other. It is often assumed that second-time mothers need less support than first-timers – 'You've done it all before; you'll be fine' is a common remark made to women who already have a child. This can make asking for help more difficult. In fact, many second-timers who did not seek help with their first baby, have more confidence to ask for help this time, and can more openly acknowledge their difficulties in the past.

Teenage and young mothers

Young mothers face very specific issues:

+ these pregnancies are often unplanned
+ the mother may not have the full support of the father
+ she may face housing and financial hardship
+ isolation from her friends and envy of their more carefree lifestyle.

It can be very daunting for a young mum to join a group where some of the women could be old enough to be *her* mother. The facilitator needs to be aware of this and encourage the young mother to participate as much as possible. It is also conceivable some prejudice may be displayed, and this must be challenged while acknowledging each individual has the right to her opinion.

Are fathers included?

In the majority of cases it is the mother who is primary carer of the baby, especially during the first few months. However, if the father is the main carer, he may also welcome the support of a group. Men in this role can also suffer PND-type symptoms brought on by loneliness and isolation and a dramatic lifestyle change.

It can be daunting to be a lone man in a group of women, and inevitably group dynamics will be affected.

+ Will the women be inhibited by male group member(s)?
+ How might the man react if the women were critical of their male partners?
+ How can the facilitator ensure the group does not become a gender war with a defensive atmosphere?

Positive outcomes include:

+ an opportunity for more understanding between the sexes
+ increased respect for a different viewpoint, which could strengthen individual relationships.

Group size

+ Eight to 10 participants is ideal. This number is large enough to generate a broad range of discussion and views, and yet small enough for everyone to have some space to contribute.
+ Larger groups may find it more difficult to bond and individuals can get 'lost'. It is all too easy for several people to talk at once and the group can split into factions.
+ Groups of less than five are unlikely to be cost-effective. Although small groups can promote more intimate sharing, the more reserved participant might find this intimidating.
+ A prior booking system will help regulate group size, although it may be impossible to confirm exact numbers until the first session. This may mean that occasionally groups are larger or smaller than anticipated, and the facilitator must be flexible in her approach to ensure the group is managed appropriately.

Crèche facilities
+ A crèche enables women with an older child to attend.
+ Two rooms will be required, which will influence the choice of venue and increase the budget.

Social and cultural diversity
The group may include women from different cultural and ethnic backgrounds with which the facilitator is unfamiliar, and she must demonstrate acceptance and respect for the variety of values within the group. The common experience of motherhood can draw women together, acting as a bridge across cultural and social divides. Diversity within the group, therefore, can offer an enriching experience that honours difference and the opportunity to appreciate and learn about other cultural traditions.

Some women from ethnic minorities may face added tensions between traditional and western values, and may benefit from a safe environment in which to explore these issues, which may be too controversial to explore within the family.

Other women may be residing in this country on a temporary basis due to work commitments. For women living away from their homeland, the postnatal period can be a particularly lonely time, and the lack of family support may be keenly felt.

Even within the UK, cultural, educational, social and class differences may be evident and need to be addressed. Although the facilitator will act in a non-judgemental manner, prejudice between group members may emerge. *See* Chapter 4 for discussion on dealing with conflict within the group.

Individuality
Although some differences, as described in the previous section, may be obvious, it is also important to respect individuality among women who, on the face of it, may be similar. Cultural, educational, social and class similarities may mask very different attitudes and values. A group of white, apparently middle-class, women can reveal as wide a diversity in outlook and mindset as a mix of cultural backgrounds. The facilitator must ensure she does not make assumptions based on outer appearances, and demonstrate appreciation for individuality.

Venue
The choice of venue will influence the 'feel' of the group. Where possible, the following can be taken into account.

Accessibility of the building
+ Is the venue on a bus route?
+ Is there adequate car parking?
+ Is there space to 'park' prams, pushchairs, and so on?
+ Is there a lift if the room is not on the ground floor?

The room

+ Small enough to encourage intimacy, but large enough to accommodate the paraphernalia that accompanies babies.
+ Is the atmosphere cheerful or dreary?
+ What is the seating like – utilitarian or comfortable?
+ Room temperature – is the heating easily regulated and can windows be opened?
+ Flooring – carpet creates a cosier atmosphere, but must be clean
+ How private is the room? If it is overlooked, this may inhibit free flowing conversation and participants may feel self-conscious breast-feeding.
+ Is the kitchen nearby?

What else is going on in the building?

How sound proof is the room? These groups can be noisy: when one baby starts to cry, others often come out in sympathy! A yoga class next door may not appreciate the sounds of crying babies.

What needs to be provided?

+ Tables for nappy changing, changing mats, emergency supplies of wipes and nappies.
+ Mats for babies to lie on the floor.
+ Toys to amuse babies.
+ Facilities to heat bottles or baby food.

And for the mothers:
+ Refreshments – tea, coffee, fruit juice, herbal tea.
+ Jugs of water to keep up fluid intake.
+ Tissues in case of high emotion.
+ A welcome smile from the facilitator!

Room rental

Charges can sometimes be negotiated if mutual benefit can be recognised: for example, basing a group at the local gym or leisure centre may encourage the participants to join and use the facilities.

These considerations will provide the best possible venue, but sometimes compromises have to be made on grounds of availability and cost. Although the physical space is important, the emotional space created by the facilitator is critical to a successful outcome.

Advertising

It is likely that a limited budget will be available for advertising and so every effort must be made to ensure it is as cost-effective as possible.

Advertising material

A poster campaign is probably the most inexpensive way to publicise the group. To ensure the poster stands out, make it as eye-catching as possible.

+ Use brightly coloured paper or white paper with coloured writing and logo.
+ Make sure the font is friendly and legible.
+ Keep a balance between illustration and writing.
+ Give two or three key points of information only.
+ Include contact details (telephone number, email address and website).

Other points to take into account

+ Laminated posters last longer.
+ A4 posters can be reduced in size for a wider distribution.
+ Leaflets provide more detail and can include a booking form.

Where to advertise

+ GP surgeries and health centres.
+ Antenatal and postnatal groups and classes.
+ Libraries.
+ Village and community centres.
+ Leisure centres.
+ Swimming pools.
+ Local shops.
+ Baby changing rooms in supermarkets and department stores.
+ Local newspaper, parish magazine or directory.
+ Magazines and newsletters advertising services and activities specifically for parents and children.

Connections made during the research stage will provide further opportunities to liaise and advertise with local groups.

Other points to consider

+ Do not rely on one method of advertising. Different types of advertising displayed in a variety of venues will ensure the message is received on a number of occasions and will yield the greatest response.
+ Posters delivered personally to chosen venues are most likely to be displayed, and discussion with the venue manager provides a further opportunity to promote the group
+ Check to ensure the advertising material has been displayed!

The most effective method of advertising is, of course, word of mouth, but this takes time to build up. In the meantime, other ways of promoting the groups must be actively pursued.

Group monitoring

Groups need to be monitored to measure their effectiveness and to assess the outcome of the aims and objectives. This evidence will influence future funding decisions. Audit information, collated by the facilitator, and evaluation feedback gathered from the participants combine to produce a report that covers the following.

Attendance

✦ Recording attendances provides ongoing feedback of group progress. If there is a significant reduction in numbers in the second week, or if attendance tails off as the weeks go by, a review is vital!

✦ Absences and reasons for absence can be noted and taken into account when assessing the success of the group: for example, a chicken pox outbreak could significantly effect numbers.

✦ Occasionally someone comes to the first session and then does not return. It may be that the group is not suitable for their needs but, if anyone misses a week, it is advisable to make contact. Sometimes a missed session can make it difficult for the woman to come again if she is shy or doesn't know anyone else in the group. Encouraging the woman to return while not applying pressure is a delicate balance.

✦ The register can also provide comparisons between groups and a variation in attendance may occur depending on the venue, the time of day of the group, or the facilitator. This information can then be analysed to aid future planning.

✦ When the group ends, a calculation can be made to work out the attendance rate: calculate as a percentage the number of actual attendances against potential attendances. This figure is one way of measuring and comparing the group outcome.

Contact list

With everyone's permission, contact information can be distributed among all participants, giving them an easy way to keep in touch between sessions. It has also sometimes been surprising for the women to discover that they live near each other without being aware of it. Landline, mobile numbers and email information eases communication.

Client information sheet

The following information provides useful data on service users that will aid future planning.

✦ How did you hear about the group?
   This information will demonstrate the effectiveness of the advertising strategy and may influence the advertising budget for future groups.

✦ Details about mother and baby.
   Details about mother, the baby's age and number of children will give background information about family relationships.

✦ Housing and work.

This information will give some indication about the socio-economic status of the participants, and will highlight anyone new to the area who may be feeling isolated.

✦ Support.

Lack of support can be a major factor in the onset of PND. Assessing the level of support, where this support comes from and suggestions for further support, can highlight gaps and identify areas of need.

✦ Pregnancy history and birth experience.

This information may influence how the woman is feeling at present. A difficult pregnancy and traumatic birth may colour how she feels about herself and the baby. These questions also give the mum the opportunity to reflect on these experiences and may trigger the need to talk through any residual anxieties. Talking in the group can be a healing experience and enable her to work through negative thoughts and fears.

Group evaluation

Evaluation tools need to be in place to assess the outcome of the group and whether the aims have been achieved. A robust method of measuring these outcomes will provide concrete evidence and data when future funding decisions have to be made.

Measurement of mental and emotional health

Gathering evidence on how the group affects the participant's mental and emotional health and well-being in her transition to motherhood is not an easy task. Screening questionnaires may be used at the beginning and end of the group and the scores compared. The following may be considered suitable.

✦ The EPDS has been widely used by health visitors and GPs to detect the onset of PND.[2]

✦ The CORE (Clinical Outcomes in Routine Evaluation) system was launched in 1998 and was developed for use by mental health services, in particular primary care counselling services.[3] Clients complete a questionnaire at the beginning and end of therapy and scores can be compared.

As discussed in Chapter 2, women at this life stage can have difficulty in disclosing any negative feelings that might indicate they are struggling or not coping in any way. They may not feel comfortable in completing a formal assessment questionnaire or, if they do, their answers may not reflect the true picture. Indeed, if these tools are used at either end of the group, their final scores may turn out to be higher than their originals. This discrepancy would indicate that women felt safer to reveal their true feelings at the end of the group and were also perhaps more aware of and in touch with their feelings. Although this would be a constructive therapeutic outcome, these results may be viewed adversely by those responsible for funding decisions unless careful explanations are given.

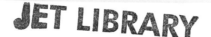

Evaluation form

An evaluation form at the end of the group is a simple and anonymous way of gathering data directly from the participants. Include:

✦ reasons for attending
✦ what was liked most and least
✦ any learning that has taken place
✦ comments on topics discussed
✦ suggestions for different topics
✦ an 'any other comments' space for more individual responses.

Storage of records

Confidential records need to be securely stored in a fireproof, lockable filing cabinet or cupboard.

Ongoing community liaison

Fostering good relationships with local health professionals and providers will help in establishing a group, and maintaining this contact can create opportunities for a collaborative and holistic approach beneficial to all.

Summary of what needs to be covered in the detailed planning stage.

■ Decide target group.
■ Arrange venue.
■ Plan how group will be monitored.
■ Set up group evaluation system.
■ Coordinate ongoing liaison with local health providers.

BOX 3.2 Detailed planning summary

References

1 Yalom ID. *The Theory and Practice of Group Psychotherapy.* 5th ed. New York: Basic Books; 2005.
2 Cox J, Holden J, editors. *Perinatal Psychiatry: use and misuse of the Edinburgh Postnatal Depression Scale.* London: Gaskell; 1994.
3 www.psyc.leeds.ac.uk (accessed 28 July 2007).

CHAPTER 4

Managing the group

This chapter concentrates on the skills required to manage a postnatal support group. Whereas the previous chapter concentrated on building the external structure, this chapter focuses on the group's internal workings and emotional structure. The philosophy and values of the group are created and practised by the facilitator, who plays a key role in the success of the group process. This chapter explores the responsibilities and skills required to manage and contain the issues brought to the group by the participants.

Group philosophy

The group provides a forum for women to discuss how they are coping with all the changes a new baby brings. Women have chosen to attend – they have not been referred or prejudged as not coping or needing help in any way. The decision to attend is an empowering one, which the group philosophy reinforces.

- A happy and emotionally healthy mother has the best chance of raising a happy and emotionally healthy child.
- There are many styles of parenting, rather than one rigid course.
- The group encourages each mother to find her own path, and to tune in and respond to her baby's needs and wants.

BOX 4.1 Values underpinning the group

One of the main reasons for attending is to meet others in a similar situation. The need to be around other women is strong at this life stage, and even those who perceive themselves as self-sufficient may feel the need to reach out to make contact with others. Women used to working or with no family nearby may feel isolated and lonely in the early months, and need to find and build a new support network.

The facilitator

The facilitator's personal qualities, skills and experience will have a direct impact on the atmosphere of the group, and will play a significant role in the group's success. She balances offering a warm and friendly relationship with the participants, while at the same time maintaining safe boundaries. She remains neutral and steady when potentially contentious and emotional issues are explored.

At the first session the participants will be appraising the facilitator, as well as each other, and will decide whether or not to return. If the facilitator creates a warm and accepting atmosphere and genuinely treats each group member with sensitivity and care, they are more likely to feel safe and engage in the group process.

Roles of the facilitator
+ To clarify aims and objectives of the group.
+ To create a safe environment for sharing of thoughts and feelings.
+ To enable discussion and maintain group focus.
+ To preserve safe boundaries within the group.
+ To be equally available to all group members.
+ To respect individual opinions.

Personal qualities of the facilitator
The facilitator acts as a role model to the group, and needs to be able to demonstrate the following qualities:
+ a warm, welcoming yet safe and containing approach
+ a non-judgemental and respectful attitude
+ a steady, consistent manner
+ care and empathy to all participants while being sensitive to individual need
+ ability to treat everyone equally
+ flexibility in approach and confidence in reacting to unpredictable situations
+ ability to tolerate and honour strong emotions in others
+ a good memory for names of mothers and babies ensures everyone feels valued
+ a sense of humour that retains a sense of balance while not diminishing problems.

■ A counselling qualification will ensure experience in counselling and communication skills.
■ Experience of groupwork, both as a facilitator and a participant.
■ Awareness of teaching approaches and learning methods.
■ Knowledge of human development, especially of this life stage and the accompanying mental health issues.
■ Good organisational and administrative skills.

BOX 4.2 Desired experience of facilitator

Limits of the facilitator

To facilitate is to enable, to assist, to make possible, to ease. The facilitator is not the expert, the adviser, the specialist, the authority, but will encourage women to make their own decisions. Nevertheless, the facilitator must remain aware that some of the group may project their own needs on to her, and expect and consider her to fulfil this 'expert' role. Any views, comments or opinions she makes, may carry undue weight and authority to the more needy mother wanting to 'get it right' and please. The facilitator must ensure she is not seduced or flattered into acting in this way, and instead work towards empowering individuals to find their own path.

Reflection

The facilitator's reflections on the ongoing progress and process of the group can form the basis for more formal supervision.

Consider:
- how does the group 'gel'?
- main themes of the session
- equal chance to speak?
- anyone giving cause for concern?
- the emotional level and tolerance of the group?
- what was 'unsaid'?
- facilitator's subjective assessment
- facilitator's response to material discussed.

BOX 4.3 Facilitator's reflections

Donald Schon has highlighted the role and usefulness of reflection.[1] He differentiated between 'reflection-in-action' and 'reflection-on-action'.

Reflection in action

The session may need to be adjusted to take account of the mood in the room:
- if it seems important to continue with an existing subject area, other issues may be postponed
- if discussion is not flowing, the facilitator may need to re-energise the group. A brainstorming exercise, initiating pairs discussion or taking a five-minute rest while everyone moves position in the room can bring a new perspective and increased energy.

Reflection on action

This takes place later when the facilitator will:
- reflect on how individuals are participating and interacting
- note how topics are received by the group to assess if any changes need to be incorporated for future groups.

Supervision

Counsellors in the UK are used to attending regular supervision to support their work with individual clients. It is a requirement of the British Association of Counselling and Psychotherapy (BACP) that all counsellors, psychotherapists, trainers and supervisors 'have regular and ongoing formal supervision/consultative support for their work'.[2]

While supervision may not be a requirement for other health professionals, it is a valuable exercise to regularly review work undertaken, and provides an opportunity to 'step back' and gain a different perspective through discussion and feedback from a colleague, who is often more experienced.

Theoretical background to the group

The theory underpinning the group is provided by the person-centred model of counselling. In the 1930s and 1940s Carl Rogers, the American psychologist and therapist, developed a new, non-directive way of working in reaction to the analytic approach of the time. Rogers believed that 'the client knows best. It is the client who knows what is hurting . . . and it is the client who knows how to move forward.' The counsellor 'enables the client to make contact with his own inner resources, rather than to guide, advise, or in some other way influence the direction the client should take'.[3]

Rogers held a very positive and optimistic view of humanity, and believed that we all have an innate drive for growth. In the same way that plants need certain conditions to thrive – for example, the right amount of light, water and warmth – Rogers believed it possible and indeed almost inevitable for people to grow therapeutically if the right conditions are provided.

- **Congruence:** being genuine and real, with no façade. This approach promotes collaboration and equality. If the counsellor can be herself, the client is encouraged to follow suit and also be 'real'.
- **Unconditional positive regard:** being accepting and non-judgemental of the client as a person. This encourages the client to confront parts of themselves that they find unacceptable in the knowledge they will not be criticised or rejected.
- **Empathy:** the counsellor is able to put her own feelings and thoughts to one side in order to understand what it is like to experience the world from the client's viewpoint. When she can communicate this understanding to the client, the client feels less alienated and isolated.

BOX 4.4 The core conditions for growth

It may initially seem deceptively simple to provide these core conditions and so promote therapeutic growth and development, but in practice it is a challenge to be able to do so to each and every client at all times. The person-centred counsellor strives to achieve this, and has to work to incorporate these conditions into the rest of her life and not just in the therapy room.

If the facilitator can adopt this framework and offer these conditions to all participants they, too, are likely to feel valued and grow in confidence and self-esteem.

Skills for groupwork

Good listening and communication skills are essential for any kind of therapeutic work, and the facilitator will need to be proficient in counselling and communication skills to encourage individuals to open up and explore topics and feelings.

Helpful counselling skills
Minimal encouragers

Minimal encouragers are the little words and phrases often used unconsciously to encourage others to keep talking: umm, Oh I see, right, I understand, OK. Non-verbal minimal encouragers include nodding, facial expression and leaning toward the talker.

Eye contact

Eye contact between talker and listener builds a connection. Whist eye contact is straightforward in a one to one situation, it is also important in a group situation when it may be more daunting to speak out. Babies easily create distractions and it may not be possible for everyone in the group to listen in a concentrated way. It is therefore very important for the facilitator to focus on the talker and not be diverted by other noises or activities, which are going on at the same time.

Mirroring

The art of mirroring, also known as reflecting, is to repeat back a key word or phrase that the client has used, which enables the client to hear again for themselves what they have just said. By repeating the exact word or phrase, the talker realises how carefully you are listening and how much you want to understand. Mirroring also keeps the talker focused on the topic of conversation, which again can be useful if the mother becomes distracted by her baby mid-sentence.

Summarising

Summarising, also known as paraphrasing, helps condense a story down, and focus on the meaning and feelings behind the words. For example, one of the group may have talked about her struggle with her baby's colic during the week and the facilitator may summarise by saying: 'It sounds as if you've been feeling very anxious that you have not been able to comfort Tom in the evenings.' This allows the woman to explore further her feelings, rather than going into coping strategies. It encourages individuals to stop and think about what is going on for them, and helps clarify and focus issues that may be muddled and unclear.

Open questions

Open questions begin with how, what, where and when, and will aid discussion. Phrases such as 'Tell me about' and 'In what way' will further focus on specific detail rather than on generalities.

Challenging

Challenging encourages the individual to take a step back and consider a different way of looking at themselves. In the group context, a mother may lack confidence in her abilities and feel that she is failing in her role. Rather than dismissing her viewpoint, the facilitator will invite the mother to examine what might be going on for her, and encourage her to focus on what she is able to do rather than what she is unable to do.

Techniques to aid discussion

Depending on the individual, joining a group can be exciting or daunting, and the facilitator needs to have a range of techniques available to encourage individual involvement and to keep everyone's interest engaged. The following techniques promote dialogue and participation.

Prompt questions

'Think back to your pregnancy and tell me what you thought it would be like at this stage . . . and what is it actually like.'

'What extra tasks have you taken on in this new role of mother?'

'Which relationship has changed most since the birth of your baby?'

'When you think back to your childhood, what instantly comes to mind?'

'Tell me any feelings you have experienced since the birth.'

'What do you like/what do you not like . . . about being a mother?'

By asking a very broad question and throwing it open to the group, the women can respond in a very general way. It is important to emphasise that there are no right or wrong answers, but that every response merits understanding.

Brainstorming

Brainstorming on a whiteboard or flipchart is a useful way of 'kick-starting' a discussion. The facilitator poses a question to the group and records all answers. The focus remains on the board and not on individuals, which makes this technique less exposing than direct discussion and participation, and is particularly suitable in the first few sessions. All contributions are noted without judgement or explanation, and the emphasis is on gaining as wide a range of answers as possible.

Brainstorming is an effective way of collecting a large number of views, feelings and issues together in a short time. Once these have been recorded, a more in-depth discussion of issues and themes can take place.

Working in pairs or small groups

Discussion in pairs or a small group of three to four can work well, and may be especially appropriate in these circumstances:

+ it helps forge individual connections in the early sessions
+ in a large group when everyone has lots to contribute and some of the input may be 'lost' owing to time constraints
+ in a group of quiet and reserved women who find it difficult to speak in the main group, and who may be more comfortable talking in small groups
+ in a group that includes some noisy babies, which may make a discussion within the whole group impractical
+ to diffuse the impact of a dominant character who might take over the group.

Each sub-group can then report to the main group and the facilitator can identify common themes. If this method is used regularly, the facilitator must encourage everyone to move around and talk with a variety of participants to avoid cliques forming, which may reinforce tension between individuals. However, if this technique is over used, it may impair bonding within the larger group.

Handouts

Handouts are essential in most types of learning groups, and are also worth considering for this group. A pack containing information about the course content with supporting handouts may be a useful addition. However, it is important to strike the right balance between a social group and an educational course, and this group falls in between. A learning pack may create a rather formal approach, which could evoke memories of schooldays and be off-putting for some women. On the other hand, individual information sheets and handouts can easily get lost or mislaid, or even chewed by the baby before they even leave the room!

The Appendices outline the main questions for each session and the handouts. Each group member could be given a copy of these to enable her to continue to think about the issues or to introduce the topic to her partner.

Paper and pen exercises

These exercises can provide a useful insight, but the success of this type of exercise depends on practicalities. Although women are very competent at multi-tasking, it is not easy to think and write while feeding a baby or soothing a fretful infant.

Written exercises can have a more powerful effect than a group discussion, and some women may fear they will reveal too much of themselves. Seeing words in black and white can throw up strong emotions and there may be a reluctance to participate. Contributing to a discussion is a matter of choice, whereas a written exercise may feel more of a pressure. For these reasons, this technique is most useful towards the end of the group, when everyone feels most secure.

Of course, it must be always be made clear that the information is for the individual's use alone, and it is up to each person to decide how much she is happy to reveal in subsequent group discussion.

Group process
Before the first meeting

The contact the facilitator has with individuals before the group begins plays an important part in setting the scene for the coming group. Prospective participants may have been in touch by telephone, email or personal contact to find out more details about the group.

If a booking system is in place, information giving time, dates, venue, directions, and so on, will have been sent out. Individuals may have been in touch with queries or to seek reassurance or guidance: 'Will it be OK to feed my baby during the meeting?', 'I'll have to leave early to collect my son from pre-school – is that alright?'

All initial contact sets the scene for the group and prospective participants will be using this information to help them decide if it is likely to be the sort of group they will feel comfortable in attending.

The first session

The first meeting of any group is very significant: it is different from all other sessions as it sets the ambience for the group. The facilitator takes the lead in setting the scene, and will work actively with the group to build a safe and caring environment, which is so vital for the group's cohesion and success. Participants will evaluate the facilitator, weigh up the other participants, assess if this particular group will meet their current needs, and ultimately decide whether or not they wish to continue in future weeks.

Room preparation

It is important that the room is ready before participants begin to arrive, and the facilitator needs to allow plenty of time to arrange the chairs and ensure refreshments, changing facilities, and so on are ready, so that she is on hand to greet each participant as they arrive. Although punctuality can be difficult with a new baby and late arrivals are likely, the facilitator must also be prepared for early arrivals. Anxiety about being late can mean arriving extra early, which may interrupt last-minute preparations, leaving the facilitator feeling rather fraught and ill-prepared herself. If the facilitator is relaxed, friendly and prepared, this will pave the way for the mothers to feel cared for and welcome.

Tasks to build a safe setting
Welcome

The facilitator welcomes the group and introduces herself.

Introductions

As an ice-breaker invite individuals to contribute to the introductory round in one of the following ways:
+ each woman introduces herself and her baby
+ divide into pairs and choose an unknown partner. Spend a few minutes finding out about each other and then introduce the partner (and baby) to the whole group. Be clear that this is not a memory test!

✦ Distribute labels for the names of mothers and babies to help everyone to get to know each other.

It is important that the women interact with each other as soon as possible. A light-hearted introductory exercise quickly raises the energy level of the group and creates a more relaxed atmosphere.

Outline of the group
✦ Give a brief history of the group and how it came into being.
✦ An outline of the weekly topics.
✦ The style of the group – highlight the differences from other groups. The word 'psycho-educational' is a mouthful, but may clarify how this group varies from social or 'baby focused' groups the mothers may already attend.
✦ Many women attend with the purpose of meeting others in a similar situation. Although the social aspect is very important, the group also offers an opportunity for women to learn about themselves.
✦ Emphasise that this is not a 'drop-in' group, and most will be gained if participants can attend every session.

Disclosure of personal information
The birth of a baby naturally evokes thoughts and memories of the mother's own childhood, and part of the work of the group is to encourage women to reflect on how their own parenting will be influenced by past experience.

There will be an invitation within the group to explore personal issues, but each woman can choose how much or how little she reveals. As previously mentioned, the sharing of information often grows as a more comfortable atmosphere is established.

Making a contract
Agree a contract with the group. This is an agreement to which everyone can contribute and then agree to abide by. When asked, the first suggestion from the group will often be a confidentiality agreement. This is an essential foundation on which to build a safe environment, and the group will not feel safe if it is not made explicit at the earliest opportunity. Although women are able to talk outside the group about what they have learnt, any personal information discussed must not be disclosed outside the room.

Confidentiality offered by the facilitator
The facilitator must think carefully about the level of confidentiality offered and make this clear to the group at the outset, so that everyone is aware of the position. Confidentiality issues will be informed by the health professionals' code of ethics and the working environment. It is unlikely that total confidentiality is feasible or ethical, and the facilitator must be clear about the circumstances when confidentiality would be broken and the course of action to be taken.

Suggestions for what could be included in a contract:
- confidentiality
- support
- respect
- giving each other space to talk
- not interrupting when another is speaking.

BOX 4.5 Making a contract

Housekeeping
- ✦ Agree dates and times. Negotiate dates to maximise attendance, taking account of bank holidays or school terms, but bearing in mind it may be impossible to accommodate everyone.
- ✦ Groups will always start and finish on time.
- ✦ Any other practical information, e.g. car parking, storage area for prams.
- ✦ Ask for permission to compose a list of contact numbers for distribution within the group. The women can then be encouraged to contact each other if a week is missed and to catch up on the discussions.

Time spent at the first session creating a safe setting will contribute to a firm foundation for future weeks. Other advantages include:
- ✦ it gives the group a chance to settle
- ✦ it provides the first opportunity to make connections with others
- ✦ creating a relaxed atmosphere will help sooth anxious mothers, who may be worried about how they or their child will cope
- ✦ boundaries, which everyone can own, are agreed jointly.

Group dynamics

Tuckman's theory of group development is probably the most well known. He identified four stages:[4]
- ✦ **forming:** the initial stage when the group comes together and the individual decides if they want to participate and continue
- ✦ **storming:** a stage of conflict when the group confronts and acknowledges differing viewpoints
- ✦ **norming:** when the group agrees ground rules and an acceptable format
- ✦ **performing:** the stage when the group is working at full potential.

In relation to the proposed postnatal support groups:
- ✦ the facilitator initially forms the group and offers a model of functioning
- ✦ storming does not always occur, as women have often come along with the prime intention of meeting others and forming new friendships. In effect, this means women are more likely to be inclusive rather than confrontational with each other. Storming may be delayed until much later when the group has formally ended and informal contact continues

+ norms do have to be established and, while the facilitator can offer a model, the group will decide upon its own norms. This is a collaborative stage in which the facilitator can participate but not direct. The norms established will shape the direction of the group
+ performing occurs when norms have been negotiated and agreed.

Early group responses indicate what is acceptable and unacceptable. For example, if an individual becomes upset at the first session, the response of the rest of the group will set the scene for future emotional reactions. They may respond with empathy and support, and so feel encouraged to disclose and express their own inner emotions. Or the group may respond with awkwardness and embarrassment, leaving the individual feeling criticised or judged. This means that different groups will be able to explore different areas and issues, and what is acceptable in one group may be taboo in another. In general, the norms of the group will determine:

+ how honest and open individuals can be
+ the level of emotion acceptable within the group
+ the degree of empathy shown to each other
+ how much self-disclosure is safe
+ the intimacy of the group.

As well as acting as a role model, the facilitator will:

+ listen and either respond directly to the person speaking or throw the topic open to the group
+ observe the reactions of the rest of the group
+ notice who does not contribute and wonder why that might be.

As the group becomes more secure, individuals become more willing and comfortable in exploring sensitive areas, and these topics will often arise as the group is more established.

Barriers to listening to each other

Any support group encourages the participants to learn from each other, and the facilitator will model active listening skills, which the group will hopefully observe and reproduce. However, barriers can arise that may inhibit or interfere with the listening process:

+ distraction by something else going on in the room
+ preoccupation with the baby's needs
+ attention wandering owing to sleep deprivation
+ worry about matters outside the group – finance, relationships, family issues
+ the mother feeling overwhelmed herself, meaning she has no capacity to hear other issues
+ denial and avoidance of painful material.

Managing the group process

The group case study in Chapters 5 to 10 charts the development of a group and illustrates some of the issues that commonly arise. The facilitator needs to be able to manage the dynamics and emotional responses from the group, and be aware of areas that could create tension between participants.

Managing difference

The factor that unites the group is that all participants have recently given birth and are adjusting to change. When individuals within the group feel understood and accepted by their peers, a sense of cohesion and support develops. However, despite their common experience, the participants may have very different backgrounds that may influence how the group progresses. Differences that may emerge include:

+ socio-economic status
+ housing
+ education
+ relationship status
+ religion.

A group that embraces different backgrounds can be enriching for all participants and lead to a greater understanding and acceptance of each other's beliefs systems and values. However, prejudice among individuals may become obvious and have a potentially destructive impact on the group.

Other more subtle differences relate to social standing and class. Michael Argyle argues there has never been a classless society and that, while sociologists and government statistics measure class by occupation, the public tend to judge class by accent, appearance, where people live, as well as education and income.[5] He concludes that health – physical and mental – and happiness are affected by social class, with the working classes faring worse than middle or upper classes. He suggests working-class life produces a greater level of stress with less effective coping strategies, causing people to feel more vulnerable and so more prone to depression. Although postnatal depression knows no barriers, socio-economic factors can play a part.

Argyle also links self-esteem with education, which traditionally has been more valued by the middle-class population. Attending a group can be daunting and, if self-esteem is low, it may be too challenging to take the opportunity to attend, and so the group may attract women who ordinarily have more confidence and who are better placed to put strategies in place to help themselves.

For many couples, the birth of a child signals a happy time in their relationship. However, this is not always the case and pregnancy and birth can create difficulties between partners. Relationships are discussed at length during the course, and the facilitator must be sensitive to the variation in experience and not make any assumptions. She needs to demonstrate respect for different views and remain neutral at all times, ensuring she does not, even unwittingly, make tactless or inconsiderate remarks. The group will inevitably be appraised by the participants and recommended

(or not) to others. Labels of 'cliquey' or 'snobby' will damage the group's reputation and could easily put off other potential participants.

Every attempt must be made to make the group as appealing and inclusive as possible, and so attractive and accessible to all new mothers.

Different personality traits

Any group will attract an assortment of personalities, which will influence the direction the group takes.

- Optimist and pessimist.
- Over-talkative, opinionated.
- Persistent attention seeker.
- The one who wants to take over and run the group.
- Joker who makes light of all issues.
- Quiet, shy person who has difficulty talking in a group.
- Expert mother with a solution for every problem.
- Emotionally expressive.
- Needy, lacking in confidence.
- Catastrophiser.
- Inflexible or intolerant.

BOX 4.6 Common personality traits

The facilitator may become aware of unspoken tensions arising between participants, and must ensure she does not collude in any scapegoating that may occur.

The facilitator will always wonder what lies behind external behaviour. For example, the persistent talker may be desperately lonely, while the joker may need to hide her depression with laughter. If judgement can be suspended in an attempt to understand, the individual may be able to talk about her anxieties and find ways of managing them.

Facilitator's responsibility to individuals

The facilitator must ensure she is equally available to everyone in the group and must not have favourites. The level of neediness among participants can be acute and rivalry can quickly develop if individuals feel overlooked. To minimise competition the facilitator must ensure:

- ✦ no one dominates discussion and therefore takes up an unequal amount of time
- ✦ there is equal invitation to contribute to discussion – quieter women may need to be asked directly for their contributions.

Reactions in groups can be more intense than normal, and jostling for position within the group can be reminiscent of sibling rivalry in families of origin and be equally painful to endure.

The facilitator must also be careful in how she relates to the babies.

✦ Do not single out an individual baby for their looks or abilities. Mothers are very sensitive at this stage and can feel both protective and upset by compliments and comments to other babies that might exclude their own.

✦ Hold or tend to a baby only if asked directly by the mother. While complete strangers have no inhibitions at approaching mothers with new babies and commenting, cooing and even touching the babies faces and hands, some women find this intrusive and distasteful. The facilitator must be cautious about taking any such liberties.

Managing emotions

The new mother has to navigate largely unknown territory in the early months and she often doubts her own abilities as she gets to know her baby. She may frequently question whether she is 'getting it right', and fears criticism and judgement from others. In her eyes everyone else seems to be so much more organised or efficient than her, and this fragility can result in emotions being very close to the surface. Sleep deprivation only intensifies this situation. Tears, anger, despair, depression, joy, elation abound and need to find some safe expression.

However, some participants may feel awkward or overwhelmed by an open display of feelings and may shy away from emotive subjects. The use of humour or a very brisk or positive attitude are common defences to avoid or deflect emotion. Sometimes those who outwardly appear most confident at the outset turn out to be the most defended and, in later stages, emerge as the most fragile.

The facilitator needs to demonstrate respect for all responses to emotional subjects. She also normalise feelings to safely contain them. When the emotional temperature of the group rises, she must also maintain the direction and focus of the discussion to encourage understanding of individual emotions and to explore more constructive ways of dealing with them. For example, session three, when changes in relationships are explored, can sometimes descend into a negative tirade against a particular relationship (partners and mothers-in-law seem to come in for most criticism). While off-loading in itself is cathartic, sharing and exploring effective coping strategies can move the relationship on.

Managing conflict

It is likely that the initial contract will have some reference to respect and acceptance of others' viewpoints, but nevertheless differences in opinions will inevitably arise, which the facilitator will have to manage. Many mothers are hypersensitive regarding their parenting style and can become very defensive if an opposing viewpoint is offered.

Common areas of debate include:

✦ Breast-feeding versus bottle-feeding
✦ Demand feeding versus regular feeding (e.g. every four hours)
✦ Working around baby versus baby should fit in with parents
✦ Sleep management
✦ Baby sleeps in own room versus in parents' bed

+ Controlled crying versus always respond to the baby's cries
+ Return to work versus stay at home
+ Organised versus 'go with the flow'
+ houseproud versus able to tolerate mess
+ discipline versus spoiling.

While many women are happy to take part in a free-ranging discussion, some can be rigid in their approach and unwilling to contemplate another opinion. Tension can grow and it is the facilitator's task to contain conflicting views, and remind the group that a definitive style of parenting does not exist.

The effect of the babies' presence

With around 12 babies (more if twins come along) in a room for one and a half hours, the proceedings can be unpredictable. The babies themselves will have a significant effect on what happens within the group and can dictate the level of participation of the mothers. Babies have immediate needs that cannot wait, and a rather chaotic atmosphere can ensue when it can be difficult for everyone to keep focus and concentration.

+ Babies communicate by crying – the strength of crying will correspond with the urgency of need; hunger for babies is life-threatening so noise levels can be disruptive.
+ Babies need attention – feeding, changing, playing with, amusing, carrying around.
+ If focus is lost, women may react by talking to each other rather than to the whole group. This may result in several conversations going on at once and the facilitator will need to draw the group back together again to re-focus.
+ Babies are very cute. Occasionally they become aware of each other and will, more by accident then design, play and coo with each other, which can be enchanting to watch and tends to bring discussion to a standstill.

While the babies can directly affect the progress of the session, some mothers will, perhaps unconsciously, 'use' the baby to deal with awkward or difficult topics and situations. The facilitator may notice:

+ a sudden preoccupation with the baby
+ engaging a neighbouring baby in play
+ the mother may talk to the group through her baby: for example, 'Toby doesn't like all this angry talk.'
+ an effort to keep discussion on a superficial level to perhaps 'protect' the baby from anything negative.

The baby may also facilitate change for women who want their children to have a different experience from their own:

+ a shy mother may take a risk to join the group to make friends
+ a quiet woman may be encouraged to speak out for the sake of her child

+ the baby may give the mother confidence to try new situations or activities.

Finally, babies work to their own personal time clock and arriving at the group on time can be challenging for women. Last-minute feeding and changing can make the most efficient timekeeper late and, although time boundaries are important, some leeway is necessary. Women may also be clockwatching if they have to collect older children from playschool, which may mean a messy end to the session. Again, this is unavoidable.

References

1 Schon D. *The Reflective Practitioner*. Aldershot: Avebury; 1983.
2 British Association for Counselling and Psychotherapy. *Ethical Framework for Good Practice in Counselling and Psychotherapy*. BACP. www.bacp.co.uk (accessed 25 March 2008).
3 Mearns D, Thorne B. *Person-Centred Counselling in Action*. London: Sage;1988.
4 Tuckman B. Developmental sequences in small groups. *Psychological Bulletin*. 1965; **63**: 384–99.
5 Argyle M. *The Social Psychology of Class*. London: Routledge; 1994.

PART B

The six-week programme

This section of the book outlines a programme for a six-session group and includes a case study of a typical group of women who might attend. Although the characters' personal circumstances, thoughts and feelings are representative of women at this life stage, they are not based on specific individuals.

The supporting notes provide background information and highlight issues women themselves have repeatedly raised. The notes provide evidence about the universal themes that women grapple with in the early postnatal period.

Overview of the six-week programme

The programme is designed as a whole package and maximum benefit will be gained by attendance at every session. The focus is on the mother and how she is feeling, giving women a chance to listen to each other and, even more importantly, to be heard. Each session lasts one and a half hours.

Course content

Introductory sessions		
Week 1	Expectations and reality	During the first two sessions the women begin to get to know each other and get used to this style of group. Confidence grows and trust builds as feelings are explored. Topics are fairly 'safe'.
Week 2	Roles of motherhood	
The real focus of the work		
Week 3	Changes in relationships	As the sense of safety increases, more personal topics can be addressed. Issues from the past may emerge. Support within the group for each other becomes more apparent.
Week 4	Parenting styles	
Week 5	Managing feelings	
Consolidation and ending		
Week 6	Building self-esteem	Sense of group identity has emerged and confidence has grown among group members.
		Celebration of ending and arrangements made to continue to meet beyond the group.

Chapter layout

Each of the six chapters in this part is laid out in the same way.

Outline Plan

An outline plan, which provides a framework for the group process, is included for each session. There are suggestions for a series of prompt questions, on topics relevant to this life stage, that can be put to the group to provoke thought and discussion.

The appendices at the end of the book contain the prompt questions and handouts for each session. There is not always time to fully discuss all the issues and the appendices can act as reminders of what was discussed as well as providing further areas for consideration. They can also be sent out if anyone misses a week to keep absentees updated on the group's progress.

Group case study

To bring the material alive, a group case study is included to illustrate what can actually happen within a group setting and demonstrate the very real issues explored. As the weeks progress, we observe how individuals respond to the course content, and also how life events continue to occur and impact on the women's emotional world.

It is a dynamic setting: the babies grow and change week by week, and the mothers learn new skills as they adapt to these changes and get to know their babies. As trust develops, relationships between participants develop, thus facilitating more sharing and exploration of thoughts and feelings.

The facilitator's preparations and reflections

The facilitator plays a key role in managing the group, and each session she records how she is feeling and thinking as she awaits the group's arrival, and her reflections log her responses at the end of the session group.

At times, she notes more personal feelings about the group process. While it is not appropriate for her to share this material with the group, she needs to recognise her feelings so that she can process them to ensure they do not get in the way of the groupwork.

Supporting notes

These notes give some further information about the issues that may arise at each session and highlight the most common themes and issues. The group case study illustrates how some of these themes might impact on the lives of individual women.

Organisation of each session

Each session lasts for one and a half hours. After this time the babies can become more fractious, and it is probably long enough for the woman to juggle the baby's needs and her involvement in the discussion. The groups offer a mixture of structured and unstructured time to ensure any immediate issues can be brought to the group and addressed, as well as ensuring the subject matter of the day is explored.

Check-in

From week two, a 'check-in' round, where everyone has the chance to say how they are feeling that day, is suggested. As well as being an ice-breaker, it provides a space for everyone in the group to contribute. Significant events or worries can be voiced and shared. As trust builds, the check-in may take progressively longer. While it is valuable to off-load, a balance needs to be maintained to ensure sufficient time is allotted to the main topic of the day.

Equipment

A whiteboard or flipchart (and suitable pens) for brainstorming sessions is useful, although it is important that the facilitator does not slip into 'teacher' mode.

Baby mats for the babies to lie on during the sessions and a box of baby supplies would be a welcome addition – spare nappies, baby wipes, nappy sacks, (although soiled nappies must always be removed from the room). Most women come laden with all necessary baby paraphernalia so only emergency supplies are required.

The focus of the session

Each session has a specific area to explore and discuss. The issues are all relevant to the new mother and often provoke lively discussion and debate. Initially, the facilitator may need to 'nudge' the discussion along but, as confidence grows within the group and the women interact more freely with each other, the facilitators input will reduce.

Summary and feedback

Allow about 10 minutes towards the end to summarise the main points raised. There may be some issues or questions that the group may wish to take away for further thought or discussion, and perhaps share with their partners. Any issues raised but not sufficiently addressed could also be highlighted.

It is also valuable, especially in the early sessions, to gain some feedback about the content and style of the group, to ensure their needs are being met and make adjustments accordingly.

Preparation for the next session

It is always useful to remind the group of next week's topic to enable them to give it some thought beforehand or perhaps to discuss it with their partners. A handout with an outline of the next topic would be a good reminder, but ensure it does not come across as 'homework', which may induce anxieties about past learning experiences and therefore be counterproductive.

CHAPTER 5

Session 1: Expectations and reality

The session
Aim
Facilitator introduces the group to the programme and creates an environment for open discussion. Group compares the expectations of motherhood to its reality.

Objectives
Introductions to each other and to the group ethos.
+ To begin to build a safe environment for sharing.
+ To find out what the group can offer.
+ To discuss and focus on expectations and reality of motherhood.

Welcome and introductions
See pp. 53–5 for a full account of how to manage the initial part of the first session.

Main topic
Once all the practicalities have been completed, the group can focus on the main topic of the session. Expectations and reality is a non-threatening subject area for the introductory session, to which everyone can contribute. The following question provides an opportunity for everyone to reflect on their pregnancy and to consider how their thoughts, feelings and expectations may have changed over past months.

> **BRAINSTORM THE FOLLOWING QUESTION:** Think back to your pregnancy. How did you imagine this time would be? What is it like in reality?

Although for some women the pregnancy may be a distant memory; for others it will still be very present in their minds. It may also be that feelings, thoughts and events that occurred during the pregnancy may have coloured how the mother reacted to the baby at birth, and may still be influencing her now. It is all too easy for this material to be 'lost' in the excitement and 'busyness' of the early days, and so many

women welcome the opportunity to reflect on the nine months leading up to the baby's arrival.

It is likely that birth stories will also emerge, and again this can be a cathartic experience to recount what happened to them.

Brainstorming the women's responses very quickly provides lots of material for more in-depth discussion and can reveal some shared experiences, which helps the bonding process begin within the group. The responses in Box 5.1 are taken from material recorded from actual groups.

Expectations	Reality
Positive	*Positive*
I would be the perfect mother.	Relief that the baby is healthy.
I would be able to cope and would be organised and tidy.	I bonded more quickly with my second child.
We would be the perfect family.	I didn't expect to feel so much love.
Breast-feeding would be easy and natural and good for the baby.	I'm grateful everything went well.
Mothering skills would be instinctive – I'll know what to do.	I'm calmer than I expected.
Fulfilling.	Emotionally fulfilling.
Enjoyable.	It's easier than I thought.
Wonderful.	
Smooth life change.	
Stress-free (compared with current lifestyle, job, etc).	
What shall I do all day while baby sleeps?	
I thought I would still have time for myself.	
I expected to bond instantly with my baby.	
My baby will be happy and contented.	
I read all the books to prepare myself.	
The baby will fit into our lifestyle.	
My child will be perfect.	
I hoped my husband would be aware of my needs and be helpful.	
Negative/Anxious	*Negative/Anxious*
I want to do it differently (from my parents).	I'm so tired all the time.
Everyone will expect me to cope.	Everything takes longer than I expected.
Will I love the baby?	I've no time for basic things like brushing my teeth.
I was afraid that I wouldn't be a good mother.	I'm shocked at how exhausted I feel.

Expectations	Reality
Negative/Anxious	*Negative/Anxious*
Will I cope?	I was unprepared for how much pain I would feel at the birth.
I worried that I wasn't feeling maternal during the pregnancy.	I feel traumatised by the birth.
Will I love this baby as much as the other(s)?	The birth was an assault on my body.
Will the baby spoil what we already have?	There were complications at the birth.
I was afraid of the birth.	My body is still recovering.
I had to fight to become pregnant.	Breast-feeding: is difficult, painful, embarrassing in front of others, I feel self-conscious, so much of a tie – I have no time for myself.
I expected it to be a nightmare.	
My friends all told me it would be awful.	I feel that I have failed as I couldn't breast-feed.
I worried that I would have PND (again).	I'm still trying to bond with my baby.
I was afraid of PND.	I'm unable to bond.
I was told it would be really hard work.	Why do I keep crying?
I knew I would be very tired.	I am emotionally drained.
This pregnancy was unplanned and I thought of having a termination at the beginning. I feel so guilty now.	I'm shocked at the intensity of feelings that I have for my baby.
	I feel very stressed.
	No time for housework.
	I have been diagnosed with PND.
	I've no time for my partner.
	There's no romance anymore.
	I'm too tired for sex.
	I'm trying to find my own way through.
	Too much conflicting advice.
	There's no spontaneity – everything has to be planned.
	Have I made a mistake?
	I've no confidence.
	I fear I might harm my baby.
	It's even more demanding than I expected.
	I've had to learn what to do – nothing has been instinctive.
	It's been anything but easy.
	I feel like I'm giving my all and getting nothing back.
	I feel: vulnerable, lacking in confidence, isolated, resentful, disappointed, hate, guilt, so much heightened emotion, anxious, worried, on edge.

Expectations	Reality
Negative/Anxious	*Negative/Anxious*
	This baby is threatening my lifestyle and my career.
	My family is concerned about me.
Lack of expectations	
I couldn't imagine what it would be like.	
I couldn't believe the bump would become a real baby.	
There will be no problems.	
I was so completely focused on the pregnancy, labour and birth that I didn't think about afterwards.	

BOX 5.1 Recurring themes

The material gathered during the brainstorm may generate sufficient discussion for the whole session. **However, if the group needs some further help to keep the discussion flowing, the following questions can be asked.** They cover 'big' issues that many women are glad to have the opportunity to explore.

Tell me about your birth experience

Thoughts about pregnancy and current experiences inevitably induce memories about the birth. Many women have a need to talk through their experiences. This may be the first opportunity they have been given.

+ Did you have a birth plan?
+ Did it go as you expected?
+ How do you feel now about the birth?

The birth can generate much discussion and is often still a vivid memory, whether it was a good or difficult experience. It can be useful to compare how the mother felt immediately afterwards and how she now feels about the experience some weeks on.

What about the bonding process with your baby?

Bonding is a much discussed topic around the birthing process.

+ When did you first notice you had bonded?
+ What was it like?
+ How has your relationship developed with your baby over the past few weeks?

There is often an expectation that the mother and baby will fall in love at the moment of birth. This does not always happen and mothers need to be reassured that everyone's experience is different.

How is feeding your baby going?
+ Did you make any plans on how you would feed before the birth?
+ Did it go according to plan?
+ If not, how are you feeling now?

Feeding is an emotional subject that can generate very strong feelings of distress, guilt and anger, as well as joy and contentment. Creating a space to express some of these feelings can be a release.

Ending the session

The facilitator needs to be aware of the time, and about 10 minutes before the agreed end time will draw the discussion to a close. Summing up the main points and highlighting both the similarities and the differences of the group's experience will provide further food for thought.

Distribute Appendix 1B, a poem about listening.

Give the group the following two questions to take away and think about.

How does it feel to talk through these current issues?

What is it like to have space to focus on yourself and your needs, rather than the baby?

Ask the group for feedback on the style of the session and remind them of next week's topic – roles of motherhood.

Equipment checklist

+ Whiteboard/flipchart and pens
+ Baby box (emergency supplies of nappies, wipes)
+ Baby mats
+ Refreshments
+ Tissues
+ Bowl to collect subs

Group case study 1

The case studies in this part are set in a market town in the south of England and give an account of the progression of a group over six sessions. Edith, a counsellor who works in a GP surgery, facilitates the group. Each session she notes her thoughts as she prepares for the group and records her comments at the end.

Eleven women have booked in and some basic information about them has been gathered from their registration forms.

Helen	Jack (9 weeks)
Jane	Josh (12 weeks)
Milka	Janka (5 months)
Karen	Sam and Beth (6 months)
Jo	Esther (11 weeks)
Sonita	Meenu (8 weeks), Asha, 6
Jenny	Lily (17 weeks), Matthew, 4
Caro	Danny (14 weeks), Tom, 3
Emma	Amy (18 weeks), Sophie 4, Joe 2
Natasha	Simone (16 weeks), Chris 12, Nick 10 and Mark 15, Sally, 13 (stepchildren)
Sarah	Amber (5 months)

Facilitator's preparations

10.20 a.m. Think I'm just about there. Ten minutes to go – kettle's boiling and the room is ready – plenty of changing mats if they want to lie the babies on the floor. Oh, where are the tissues, just in case. Always best to be prepared.

I've enjoyed running these groups in the past three years, but yet always feel a little on edge before everyone arrives. Starting a new group is exciting but daunting, too.

Wonder if they will all come today – 11 booked in, which is a good number. I think a couple of them attended the talk I gave to the antenatal class so there may be some familiar faces. I had a long conversation with Emma last week – she's not sure how many she will be able to attend as she has two other children – she sounded very stressed so I hope she does manage to come.

None of us knows how the next few weeks will go but that is what makes the work so interesting – we are all starting on a journey together and who knows where it will take us. It's just like motherhood – they will all make their individual journeys and I walk alongside them in these early weeks.

I could do with a coffee myself.

Suddenly the door opens 'Is this the right place?', 'Can I bring the pram inside?' We're off.

The session

Group process	Comments
About 10 minutes before the start time the women begin arrive. It takes some time for them all to settle and to make the babies comfortable.	The facilitator welcomes the women as they arrive and offers refreshments.
Some of the babies begin to fuss and need to be fed or changed. Soon the room is full of mothers, babies and all the accompanying paraphernalia that accompanies small babies.	The mothers need to be reassured that they must do whatever is needed to keep the babies happy.
Jane, Helen and Sonita have all attended the same antenatal class and so know each other a little. Jo and Natasha have recently moved to the area and do not know anyone locally. Caro and Milka also do not know anyone.	The facilitator introduces herself to the group and enquires if anyone in the group has already met.
Emma and Jenny know each other by sight from pre-school.	She then suggests everyone find a partner who is unknown to them, and to chat to each other for about five minutes; then they will be asked to introduce their partner to the group.
Much light-hearted reaction to this suggestion about still having a 'pregnancy brain' and so unable to remember anything, but reassurance that it is not a memory test. Facilitator encourages the group to settle to find a partner and soon the room is alive with chatter.	
In the middle of the introductions, Karen arrives, double buggy and massive changing bag in tow. She looks exhausted; she tells the group she has been on the go since 6.30 a.m. in an attempt to reach the group on time and was feeling very pleased with herself that she had made it, even if a little late until she realised on her 20-minute walk to the venue that she had forgotten to brush her teeth or her hair before leaving the house!	Due to each baby's sense of timing, someone is nearly always late and on this first session it is Karen.

Karen's honesty breaks the ice and she gratefully gulps down a large mug of black coffee (breakfast!). Introductions resume and the group begins to get to know each other.

When the introductions are complete, the facilitator explains the aims of the groups, agrees the contract and outlines other housekeeping issues (*see* pp. 54–5 for more details). |
Expectations and reality	The main topic of the day is then introduced.
The group responds well to the brainstorm and before long the board is filled with thoughts and feelings. The group talks about their recent experiences.	
Helen seems quietly confident, loved being pregnant, had a straightforward birth and is really enjoying her baby son. She admits to feeling tired, but accepts that it will not last forever and is very grateful for the baby's safe arrival and how 'good' he is.	

Group process	Comments
Emma contributes a lot to the discussion and is very open about her experiences after the births of her two previous children – she had PND after the birth of her second child and is anxious in case it happens again. She has come to the group as she feels she needs as much support as she can get.	Emma becomes very animated as she speaks.
Natasha confesses to feeling very new to motherhood, even though this is her third child – she has two boys (12 and 10) by a previous marriage and feels she had forgotten it all.	
Sonita can identify with Natasha as her daughter is aged six and has been at school for the past 18 months – she too feels much has changed in these six years as all her friends have passed the baby stage. Although she has strong family support, she wanted to meet other mums with babies of similar age.	Even at this stage the group seems to be comfortable and begin to interact with each other directly.
Caro says she feels much more confident this time around, compared to how she felt after her first son, now aged three. So far she feels she is coping better and hopes she will enjoy the experience more than last time, when she felt overwhelmed by her new responsibilities of looking after a child.	Some of the women are able to voice their anxieties, indicating how important these issues are for them. This openness will hopefully encourage others to share how they are really feeling.
Karen is recognisable as the joker of the group and makes everyone laugh with her tales of her pregnancy, her reaction to the news that she was having twins and her more recent exploits in trying to shop with a double buggy.	The presence of twins may mean the facilitator will have to have a more 'hands on' approach than usual!
Milka explains she was invited to the previous group but didn't feel ready to join at that stage. Milka is Slovakian and, although she has lived in the UK for 10 years, she still felt nervous about joining this type of group. However, as Janka is now 5 months, she is more confident about meeting new people.	Despite her nervousness, Milka appears friendly and open to the group.
Jo seems rather shy, although relaxes a little as the discussion gets underway. She tells the group that she moved just a few weeks before her baby was born and is still getting to know her way around. Towards the end of the introductions Esther, Jo's baby, begins to cry and, despite everything Jo tries, she is unable to comfort her. Esther's crying becomes louder and Jo becomes increasingly distressed and tearful herself, as she is worried about disrupting the whole group. Jo begins to gather up her belongings and says she will leave, but the facilitator asks her not to and acknowledges that every mother has been there at some time or other. Caro offers to hold Esther to give Jo a break and she gratefully accepts. Eventually Esther gives a loud burp and falls asleep. Jo is able to put her in her car seat.	Many new mothers worry about having to contend with a crying baby who cannot be comforted. There is a huge amount of support and empathy among the women for Jo and, in fact, this incident helps bond the group at this very early stage. Jo is able to accept help in the spirit in which it was given.

Group process	Comments
Jane is very positive about her experience of motherhood, however much of her attention is taken up being busy with her baby – feeding, winding and changing him. She doesn't seem to engage much with what is going on in the room.	
Jenny says little about herself during this first session, although listens intently to the others.	Inevitably some women are more vocal than others and it is important that the more quiet members of the group are given the opportunity to speak to ensure a division does not emerge. Everyone's experience is valuable and it is vital that the group is not dominated by one or two personalities.
Themes which generate most discussion are the birth, feeding, sleep, or lack of it, and bonding. A lively discussion continues and time passes quickly.	Initially the facilitator's role is to get the discussion moving, encouraging everyone to contribute. The facilitator needs to acknowledge differing views and demonstrate each is valid.
Feedback	
Feedback at the end of the first session is positive with the women commenting on how good it is to have some time to talk about themselves, as the focus of the past few weeks has been almost entirely on the baby. They are surprised at the commonality of feelings and experience, and seem glad to have another session booked for the following week.	The facilitator needs to be aware of the time and bring the session to a close with enough time for the group to comment on how they have found this initial session. She reminds everyone of the weekly charge and provides a bowl to collect the subs, and distributes the listening poem (Appendix 1b).
	She also asks permission to compile a contact list with everyone's details for distribution next week, and concludes with a reminder of next week's topic – roles of motherhood.
At the end of the group, Emma and Caro rush off to collect other children from pre-school, and Jane and Helen also leave promptly. The others linger and chat in a relaxed way as they gather their bits and pieces together. Even when they leave the room, they continue their conversation outside for some time.	The facilitator tidies up the room and makes herself available in case anyone wants a private word. She is aware the room is booked for another meeting that starts shortly, but is reluctant to hurry the women out.

Facilitator's reflections

✦ Good first session – everyone contributed, although the first-time mothers spoke less than the others – must ensure they have enough space next time.

✦ Reasonable cultural mix of women this time. Even within the UK we have range of backgrounds – Jo is Scottish and Caro was brought up in Devon.

+ Often I get a sense of everyone weighing each other up in the first session but the incident with Jo's baby brought the group together. The group support for Jo was really positive. If she had left in the middle of the group, I don't think she would have returned.

+ Jane was the only one who seemed unmoved by Jo's plight – she remained rather detached and self-contained. She was very involved with her baby throughout. She looked confident but maybe her focus on Josh covered up her shyness. Or maybe she was really irritated by Esther's crying. I guess time will tell as we get to know her better – if she comes back.

+ Karen puts a positive spin on everything, always seeing the funny side of things. Must ensure she doesn't take over/keep it all very light. This group aims to give time and space to all kinds of feelings – the negative and uncomfortable, as well as happy and positive.

+ Helen also paints a very rosy picture of her life at present – interesting non-verbal reactions from some of the second-time mums! – almost a smug 'you just wait' in their expressions.

+ Caro's honesty about her feelings following her older son's birth paved the way for others to be more open about how they really feel.

+ Emma came across as being quite vulnerable, with a desperate need to talk about her feelings. She could easily dominate the discussions. May need more support than this group can give?

+ Milka was clearly nervous at the beginning of the group but relaxed as the discussion got under way and contributed quite a lot, especially to the sleep debate. I wonder if her husband's family are around to give much support?

+ Jenny, Sonita and Natasha all seemed to settle in well, although they may need to be drawn out more next time. Jenny, in particular, didn't give away much about herself.

+ Interesting how the expectations of the first-time mums varies from the women who already have a child. Some of the first-timers couldn't see beyond the birth and don't seem to have given this bit much thought. It's much less of a shock second time around, although if the baby is very different, that can also cause problems

+ As usual the 'big' themes were the birth and feeding. Two emergency and one elective caesarean sections – around the national average – and a couple of the others are still recovering physically from their natural births. Helen's birth seemed enjoyable – much to the envy of some of the others. I think Jane and Natasha are the only ones still solely breast-feeding, although some of the others are doing a mixture of breast and bottle. They may need to talk more about these issues in future weeks.

+ I wonder what happened to Sarah? I'll give her a ring (phone call – she has decided not to join after all as she is shortly returning to work).

Supporting notes

The responses in Box 5.1 are consistently reported by women in the first session. Although often a group of strangers, they nonetheless have shared a common experience and are keen to understand each other, and often display sensitivity to each other's circumstances. This shared experience seems to strip away usual inhibitions, and women need little encouragement to reveal their more private thoughts and feelings.

Women can be surprised that reality is so different from what they expected. Those who expected it to be 'a nightmare' sometimes find it relatively easy, while those who thought they would take it all in their stride may struggle. Sometimes dealing with the pregnancy means little thought is given to the early postnatal months.

Many of the responses are spoken from the heart, and often reveal vulnerabilities and anxieties usually left unspoken. This first session can have a significant effect on many of the women who attend. They feel able to express their inner thoughts and feelings, and realise, most surprisingly, that others can identify with these thoughts and feelings.

The eagerness of the participants indicates a real need to talk about this momentous event and how their lives have changed forever. This discussion throws up how different reality is from fantasy. No matter how much preparation is completed beforehand – decisions about baby equipment, nursery decor, the type of nappy, and so on – the emotional impact of having a baby is frequently completely overlooked. And often, it is the emotional impact that causes most upheaval, and 3–4 months later women are still adjusting to it.

In the hurly-burly days of a new life, when there so much to do and so many new skills to master, it is all too easy to forget to ask the mother how *she* is, and how is *she feeling* and *coping*. Providing a space to talk and giving women the opportunity to off-load can be a relief. All too often, new mothers believe they are alone with these uncomfortable thoughts and feelings, and do not feel they dare reveal them to anyone else. Thoughts can quickly escalate to:

'I must be a really bad mother/person to have these feelings.'

'No one must know how I really feel; I have to pretend it's wonderful.'

'Will they take my baby away?'

These mothers need reassuring and, although the facilitator can provide some of this, they will receive most reassurance from their peers, the other women in the room. Mutual support, which can begin in the first half hour of the group, can be moving and inspiring.

Pregnancy

More often than not, the announcement of pregnancy is greeted positively: 'Congratulations', 'How lovely; you must be delighted', 'When are you due?', 'Are

you keeping well?' Sometimes the announcement is greeted with humour: 'Just you wait', 'Make the most of your freedom while you can.'

For the most part, society also looks on pregnant women with optimism and hope, although the reasons for having a baby are many and varied, including:

+ a primitive need to procreate
+ to fulfil a long-term ambition
+ to satisfy family expectations
+ to have someone to love and be loved in return
+ to carry on the family line
+ to aid an ailing relationship
+ to replace a lost child
+ to heal the past.

The woman may or may not be consciously aware of these reasons, and they may only come to light on reflection.

The strength of the woman's biological body clock should also not be underestimated. Women who had previously made a conscious decision not to have a child suddenly become aware of a nagging and growing desire when they hit their mid-30s.

The motivation to have a child may be stronger in one partner than the other, and sometimes it is the man who is keener than the woman. If the couple are able to discuss their feelings frankly and to work through any ambivalence, they are likely to be more prepared for the task of parenthood.

Common ambivalent responses to pregnancy

Not all responses to pregnancy are positive and often ambivalence is present.

The unplanned pregnancy

It may not be the right time, the right circumstances or the right partner. The father may not be around. A termination may be contemplated, and this may be a lonely time as the woman thinks about her future.

The pregnancy happened immediately

When the woman falls pregnant very quickly, the couple sometimes feel unprepared and even cheated of all that 'practice time' they were hoping for! It might feel too soon and the enormity of the decision can seem huge. They may even feel rather guilty that it was all so easy for them, especially if friends or family are having fertility problems.

A long wait to conceive

At the other end of the scale, some couples do not find it at all easy to conceive, and may have had long and intrusive fertility treatment. The goal to conceive and *be* pregnant almost becomes an end in itself, and the pregnancy may be fraught with anxiety.

A history of miscarriage

Miscarriage is common – one in four pregnancies ends this way – so it is likely that some women in the group will have suffered this loss previously, or even have a history of multiple miscarriages.

Its frequency does not reduce the pain it causes and may colour subsequent pregnancies. The woman may not allow herself to believe that this pregnancy will result in a live birth. In particular, the timing of the previous miscarriage will cause concern in the current pregnancy and be viewed as a hurdle to cross before she can relax and enjoy this pregnancy.

Previous stillbirth

Miscarriage becomes a stillbirth any time after 24 weeks gestation. The baby's birth can then be registered and a funeral can take place, which can be an important part of the grieving process.

The emotional pain of a previous stillbirth will be ever present during subsequent pregnancies, and anxiety levels are likely to increase as the birth draws closer. The woman is all too aware that a healthy pregnancy does not guarantee a healthy baby, and she will need extra support and sensitivity from professionals, family and friends at this time.

Previous termination

Memories of any previous termination may emerge at any time during the pregnancy, especially if there is the added worry of a threatened miscarriage. Feelings of guilt or regret may be strong and the woman may re-live and re-evaluate her life at that time, and the decision previously made. Again the duality of emotions – joy at the current pregnancy and sorrow about the previous pregnancy – can be confusing to handle.

Health during pregnancy

Morning sickness, backache, constipation, stretch marks, haemorrhoids, heartburn, insomnia, tiredness, varicose veins, thrush and flatulence are just some of the common delights of pregnancy, which most women find more irritating than distressing. However, persistent sickness that goes way beyond the first trimester, pre-eclampsia and gestational diabetes may all create more worry and complications during the pregnancy, and may be repeated in subsequent pregnancies.

History of eating disorders

For women who have struggled with an eating disorder at an earlier life stage, pregnancy can be a particular challenge. Anorexia nervosa and bulimia nervosa are conditions where control is important – if other aspects of life appear out of control, what is eaten is the one area that can be controlled. These conditions are often accompanied by a distorted body image. As the woman's body changes during pregnancy, past feelings of anxiety, chaos and depression may arise, causing distress to the woman, who may never have disclosed her past difficulty with food.

These ambivalent reactions to pregnancy may, in some instances, affect the

mother's relationship with the growing baby. If these feelings persist, she may feel anger towards the baby for causing her such hardship. This can be accompanied by guilt, making the woman feel completely wretched. In addition to affecting the pregnancy, this guilt can persist in the postnatal period and contribute to PND.

Such feelings may be too frightening to voice or even acknowledge during pregnancy, and are more likely to be hidden and suppressed. The safe arrival of the baby may make it possible to talk through these feelings as a way of letting them go.

At the beginning of the group, little may be known about the individual history of each participant but, as the group progresses, some of the above may come to light. The act of speaking out and being heard is affirming, and acceptance by others can have an empowering and positive affect.

Progression of pregnancy

Pregnancy lasts 40 weeks. As the mother's body prepares for birth during this time, the couple will also be working through different thoughts and feelings in preparation for the new arrival.

Pregnancy is roughly divided into three trimesters of approximately 12 weeks each, with information about the developing foetus often described according to these three stages. Joan Raphael-Leff identifies three phases, which correspond to the three trimesters, that she calls 'transformational stages', when the 'focus shifts from pregnancy to foetus to baby'.[1]

The first trimester (0–12 weeks)

Confirmation of the pregnancy can arouse a range of emotions and physical reactions, as the woman's body undergoes changes. The couple may not tell everyone their news until after the 12-week scan and when the pregnancy has become more established.

The second trimester (13–28 weeks)

The trimester when women usually feel very well: 'blooming' is often used to describe the pregnant women during his period. The pregnancy has become more real and the couple may develop a picture of a fantasy or idealised baby. This is the least anxious trimester.

The third trimester (29 weeks to birth)

Increased tiredness as pregnancy progresses, and growing thoughts and anxieties about the birth, although relief that the baby would usually now survive if born early. Final planning and practical preparations.

Approaches to pregnancy

Daniel Stern describes three patterns of attachment that begin in pregnancy and that are influenced by the woman's personal experience and history:[2]

+ **Enmeshed attachment pattern**

  The woman immerses herself completely in the pregnancy. She is likely to be very

close to her own family and increasingly identifies with her own moth/ pregnancy progresses.

+ **Dismissing attachment pattern**
  The woman attempts to keep motherhood at a distance and shows little interest in how she was mothered herself. She appears to be not very emotionally involved in the pregnancy and does not wish to talk about it.
+ **Autonomous attachment pattern**
  The middle ground: although the woman can lose herself in her relationship with her baby, and is involved and interested in her mother's experience of mothering, she also has the capacity to reflect on past experiences. She drifts between feeling and thoughts about the feelings.

Raphael-Leff has also identified three broad responses to the pregnant state:[3]

+ **The facilitator** adores being pregnant and devotes herself totally to her baby's well-being. Pregnancy is a culmination of her femininity and links her to a long line of pregnant women – her mother, grandmother, and so on. We might recognise her as an 'earth-mother' type.
+ **The regulator** sees pregnancy as a rather tedious way of getting a baby. She doesn't want the pregnancy to interfere with her life and tolerates minimal changes to lifestyle. She retains a sense of detachment from the growing baby.
+ **The reciprocator** takes the middle ground and, although may be overjoyed, she is also regretful of the changes to lifestyle the baby will produce. She is more aware of her ambivalence.

Raphael-Leff does not suggest these responses are based on personality characteristics, but on the woman's current understanding of herself; nor does she claim these are fixed responses, as they may change in subsequent pregnancies.

Stern and Raphael-Leff agree that all three styles are normal ways of adapting to the 'psychological turbulence that becoming a mother entails', to quote Raphael-Leff. Although it is helpful to be mindful of the variety of responses to pregnancy and mothering, women do not neatly fall in to a particular category. It is important for the facilitator to keep an open mind and be aware of the wide spectrum of responses, rather than labelling or 'pigeon-holing' the mother.

Women also report a significant change in their attitude to mothering after the baby is born. Some women, tending towards the regulator end of the spectrum during pregnancy may find themselves veering much more towards the facilitator mode as they fall head over heels in love with their new baby. Any unanticipated emotional reaction can be disturbing for women to acknowledge and embrace.

Domestic abuse

Although pregnancy is a happy event for many couples, this is not always the case, and in some circumstances pregnancy may trigger or exacerbate male violence. The Royal College of Midwives (RCM) recognises just how vulnerable women can be at this time and 'supports routine enquiry into domestic abuse throughout pregnancy and

the postnatal period'. If abuse is suspected, the midwife is urged 'to ask the woman explicitly but carefully and sensitively' for more information. The midwife can then provide the woman with further information or referral to an appropriate agency.[4]

The facilitator also needs to be aware of women's added vulnerability during pregnancy, and be able to provide information about local agencies offering support around issues of domestic abuse.

The birth

In late pregnancy, plans for the birth take shape. Women are encouraged to attend antenatal classes, which are run by the hospital or local midwives; alternatively, some women choose to attend private classes such as those run by the National Childbirth Trust. Yoga classes for pregnant women, where the focus is very much on the birth, are also popular.

In the last 30 years, birth has become increasingly medicalised and reliant on technology. In 2005, the RCM launched the Campaign for Normal Birth, which recognised that pregnancy and birth are normal physiological processes, and stated its commitment to work towards the reduction of unnecessary medicalisation, while giving the mother a better birth experience.[5]

The NCT, founded in 1956, also believes women should have the opportunity to have a normal birth; that is, one without induction, surgical interventions, caesarean sections or the use of anaesthesia in labour. However statistics from 2005–06 indicate natural birth is still difficult to attain:[6]

+ 46.7% of births classified as 'normal'
+ Caesarean sections 23.5%, emergency caesarean sections 14.1%, planned 9.3%
+ Induced births 20.2%
+ Use of epidural 22%
+ Instrumental births (use of forceps/ventouse) 11.1%.

The vast majority of women give birth in hospital, although in some areas birthing centres are an alternative. These centres are run by midwives and offer women the opportunity to have a natural birth. Birthing centres are not suitable for everyone and, if the woman has a history of high blood pressure, if she is expecting twins, or if there are known problems with the baby, a hospital birth will be advised. Birthing centres are popular with women and their families for offering more 'homely' care than maternity units.[7]

In April 2007, the Royal College of Obstetricians and Gynaecologists and the RCM issued a joint statement of their support for home births for women with uncomplicated pregnancies.[8] This statement recognises that birthing at home can be an empowering and fulfilling experience, where women experience less pain and have fewer interventions. Although home births currently account for only 2% of total births, it is thought that, if women were given a real choice, this would increase to 8–10%. This need for choice has been recognised in the Department of Health publication *Maternity Matters: choice, access and continuity of care* (2007), which states that by 2009 women will be able to choose how they access maternity care, the type

of antenatal care and the choice of place of birth, with home birth being a clear option.[9]

It is the provision of choice that is important. Some women will always want a natural birth with minimal interventions, while others prefer the choice and control that technology offers.

Birth preparation classes are invaluable, especially for the first-time mother, but focusing on the physical aspects of the birth can mean that little time is spent thinking about the postnatal period. At this stage, it seems almost impossible to think beyond the hurdle of the birth, which seems to become the end goal rather than a beginning.

Giving birth is the bridge between the pregnancy and mothering. It is always a memorable occasion, and many women can give detailed and vivid accounts of their baby's birth years after the event. Reactions to the birth on both the physical and emotional levels can preoccupy the mother in the early postnatal days, and may affect the bonding process.

Birth factors that may affect bonding
+ Did the birth go as planned?
+ Who was present?
+ Was the birth straightforward?
+ Any medical interventions necessary, e.g. drugs, forceps, ventouse or caesarean section?
+ Length of labour – either very speedy or prolonged.
+ Support from health professionals.

The first time a woman gives birth she has little idea of her tolerance of pain and how she will cope with it. The woman who vowed to have her baby naturally may be screaming for an epidural within the first couple of hours of labour. Conversely, the woman who thought she would accept any intervention offered may progress and deliver before she felt the need for help.

Approaches to birth
Raphael-Leff suggests the woman's approach to the birth will mirror her approach to pregnancy.[10]
+ **The facilitator** believes she must surrender herself to the labouring process in order to be reunited with her baby after the birth. The word 'surrender' evocatively suggests a relinquishment to the process. She may wish for a home birth, or at least minimum medical intervention, and will want her baby by her side at all times. An early discharge from hospital will allow her to continue to bond with her baby without interruption or intervention.
+ **The regulator** views birth as a medical event, and will accept any intervention offered that will alleviate or curtail the inevitable pain of labour. She will feel safer in hospital, but her main fear will be loss of control of her body and her feelings. Any support offered that contributes to her retaining control will be

eagerly sought. She may want some time to recover before she makes her baby's acquaintance, and may be happy to use the hospital nursery in the first few days.

✦ **The reciprocator** treats the birth as a natural process and, although may refuse the use of some drugs, she is likely to accept the more benign interventions of gas and air or a TENS machine to help with the pain. If she chooses a home birth, she will feel safer if the hospital is close by in case complications arise. She will find the birth exhilarating and be keen to meet her baby.

Some women are ecstatic in the first moments of their baby's life, and are overwhelmed by a sense of achievement and contentment, the recent of pain of labour already forgotten. Others, who have endured a long and difficult labour and been stretched to the limit – physically and psychologically – may not be in the best frame of mind to meet their new baby and show little interest in the first moments. However, many women remember:[11]

✦ the baby's first cry, which confirms his safe passage into life
✦ the feel of the baby as he is placed on the mother's belly
✦ the shift upwards to her breast
✦ the first gaze
✦ the first feed.

These can be profound moments in a woman's life, when she experiences a sense of continuity and connection with the world and with all those who have given birth before. Feelings of achievement and contentment wash over the new mother, especially if the birth experience has been positive.

Unexpected complications

For some women, the birth does not go according to plan and complications may mean an emergency caesarean section, or other unforeseen interventions. Some women may be shocked by the intensity of pain they had to endure, and feel physically and emotionally traumatised by the whole experience.Other women may still be dealing with the after-effects of the birth weeks or months later, as their bodies have still not fully recovered. Continuing pain and discomfort cloud the early postnatal period, leaving the woman cheated of the experience she had hoped for.

The premature baby

A premature birth takes place if the baby is born prior to 37 weeks gestation. These babies cause extra concern and worry, and may have to spend many weeks in the hospital's special care baby unit. Parents are encouraged to spend as much time as possible helping to care for their baby until he is well enough to be discharged. The mother may feel unprepared for the birth when the baby arrives early, and may feel guilty that she was not able to successfully complete the pregnancy.

The first-time mother will be able to devote her time there but, if the mother has other children, she will be torn between the needs of her older children and the new baby. This can be a particularly stressful time for the family and put extra strains

on everyone. Even when discharged from hospital, the couple may be advised to protect the baby from any potential health risks, and contact with other people may be limited. This can further isolate the mother and make it difficult for her to find the social support she needs.

Parents of babies born prematurely will have experienced many feelings of worry, anxiety, fear and, ultimately, relief that all is well. It may take some time for these issues to come to the surface, and they may need extra support at a later date to work through these anxieties.

The group provides an opportunity to explore the intense feelings about the pregnancy and birth experience, which may have been pushed aside by the birth celebrations.

Reality
Coming home

The length of stay in hospital after giving birth has reduced considerably in recent years, and currently a first-time mother who has had a normal delivery can expect to be discharged as early as six hours after the birth. Even women who have had a caesarean section are discharged any time from day three. Although some women view a caesarean section as an easier birth option, there is concern among health professionals that the rate of caesarean sections has risen over the past 30 years.[12] The recovery time is much longer than a natural birth, and it is likely the mother will need extra care and support in the early days – she has just undergone major surgery.

Society now seems to expect the mother to be back to normal and fit for anything within hours of giving birth. Although many women want to get home to a comfortable environment as soon as possible, the weight of responsibility can be daunting, and the first few weeks can be a particularly anxious time until some sort of familiarity of routine emerges.

This can also be quite a social time as a stream of visitors descends on the household to greet the new baby. While the couple may welcome the attention and want to share their excitement of the birth, it can also be hard work entertaining visitors, and leave them feeling exhausted.

The early days may reawaken ambivalences of the pregnancy that had previously been laid to rest – 'Am I ready for this?', 'Can I cope?' – while new anxieties can also develop, from 'Am I a good mother?' to fears around the possibilities of cot death or other health related issues.

Other cultures treat this early postnatal time differently, giving the couple time to adapt to their latest addition. In Tibetan tradition, family and friends must wait three days after a boy is born and four days after the birth of a girl before they visit. In late pregnancy, Moroccan women have their hands painted with intricate patterns using henna paste and, as long as the henna remains visible, she is exempt from all household duties, ensuring at least three weeks rest. In addition, the mother receives a stimulating massage of henna, walnut oil and kohl during her postnatal confinement. Many western women would welcome such nurturing in these early weeks![13]

The early weeks

The new mother faces a steep learning curve in the early weeks of her new baby's life:

+ meeting and getting to know her baby
+ learning how to handle him and tend to his needs
+ becoming familiar with new skills and realising that multi-tasking takes on a whole new meaning.

Within herself she also has to deal with:

+ facing her new responsibilities
+ managing the anxieties, which this unknown role brings
+ recovering from the birth, physically and emotionally.

Some women also report the 'loss' of being pregnant. These are women for whom pregnancy has been a particularly enjoyable experience and who have not quite let go of the fantasies surrounding the 'imaginary' baby.

As the weeks and months progress, the new mother will begin to grapple with these issues, and will eventually work her way through to find her own way of dealing with the new role.

The responsibility of a new baby – the unfamiliarity of looking after one so utterly dependent – can feel scary to the new parents. No matter how many books they have read, they may still feel unprepared for the enormity of what lies ahead. The gradual realisation that this role lasts forever is daunting. And yet, despite this, there is a frequent expectation that all will be well and a smooth transition to parenthood will occur as the parents take to their new roles with ease – after all they have a beautiful baby.

In reality, this can be a stressful time for many new parents as they get to grips with feeding, bathing and changing – activities that are time-consuming and not easy to master. As weeks go by, there is the never-ending desire for sleep, sleep and more sleep, as the baby dictates the pattern of the household, turning day and night upside down.

> During pregnancy, the woman prepares herself for birth, but is often unprepared for the new world of motherhood. Birth acts as the bridge between pregnancy and motherhood.
>
> 'Normal' life is suspended during the early weeks and months as the process of adjustment to motherhood begins.
>
> Women need contact with other women going through the same life stage for mutual support and understanding.

References

1 Raphael-Leff J. *Pregnancy: the inside story*. London: Karnac; 1993.
2 Stern D, Brushweiler N, Freeland A. *The Birth of a Mother*. London: Bloomsbury; 1998.

3 Raphael-Leff J., op. cit.
4 www.rcm.org.uk (accessed 23 March 2008).
5 Ibid.
6 www.birthchoiceuk.com (accessed 23 March 2008)
7 www.naturalmatters.net (accessed 23 March 2008).
8 www.rcm., op. cit.
9 www.dh.gov.uk (accessed 23 March 2008).
10 Raphael-Leff J., op. cit.
11 Stern D, *et al.*, op. cit.
12 www.rcm., op. cit.
13 Jackson D. *Baby Wisdom*. London: Hodder Mobius; 2002.

CHAPTER 6

Session 2: Roles of motherhood

The session
Aim
To explore the roles, qualities and skills a mother uses.

Objectives
+ To list all roles involved in mothering.
+ To explore skills required to carry out all roles.
+ To appreciate the diversity and complexity of the roles of motherhood.
+ To compare current role with own mother's / grandmother's role.
+ To explore how to incorporate the new roles into the rest of our life.
+ To further value ourselves in light of the above.

Check-in
+ Everyone has the opportunity to say how they are feeling today and to share anything of significance from the past week.
+ Any comments about last week – style of group, and so on?
+ Did last week's discussion provoke any further thoughts?

Main topic
Before the baby arrives it is difficult to imagine how each day will be spent. It is often thought babies sleep for extended periods, leaving the new mother with plenty of time on her hands. By this stage, the women in the group will be all too aware of the work involved in childcare, and will be growing accustomed to the many and varied daily tasks to be done. This session asks them to explore how this role will expand in the future, with the changing needs of a growing child, and how their latest role can be integrated into the rest of their life.

> **BRAINSTORM THE FOLLOWING QUESTION: What is a mother? Think of all the roles, skills and qualities required to fulfil this role.**

housekeeper	entertainer	emotional support	cook
skivvy	friend	bottle washer	gardener
car washer	nagger	disciplinarian	housemaid
nappy changer	baby cleaner	nurturer	launderer
secretary	teacher	role model	social organiser
dog walker	accountant	role model of morals/ manners	teacher of social skills
playmate	adviser	book keeper	pet carer
counsellor	nurse	shopper	guide
carer	ironer	taxi driver	chauffeur
protector	house cleaner	shopper	financial manager
educator	peace maker	diplomat	Mrs Fixit
comforter	mind reader	confidante	security giver
reassurer			

BOX 6.1 Roles of motherhood

It is interesting to note that this list includes some of the more traditional homemaking roles, which previously may have been shared when both partners have been working.

To be able to:	
juggle	prioritise
multi-task	give praise
be there physically and emotionally	split yourself
work well under pressure	be inventive
fit everything together	manage time efficiently
be a good listener	

BOX 6.2 Skills and abilities

These lists are not exhaustive, but are examples of what women have consistently reported. The roles, skills and qualities provide the growing child with a mixture of practical and emotional support. Several professions are rolled into one: carer, teacher, counsellor, adviser, entertainer, doctor, secretary, manager, coach and accountant, to name just a few. This brainstorming session highlights the many demands each woman will face, and underlines the value of this role, which is often underrated in today's society. The many roles she adopts, and the skills and qualities required, highlight how mothers give out so much to others, often leaving them little time or energy to think about themselves.

To have:	To be:	
sense of responsibility	organised	affectionate
sense of humour	playful	giving
patience	understanding	fit and healthy
empathy	loving	versatile
stamina	fun loving	methodical
tolerance	understanding	unselfish/selfless
imagination	light sleeper	motivated
	adaptable	practical
	enthusiastic	calm

BOX 6.3 Qualities

Putting the role of a mother today into context

In what way is your current role different from your mother's, or even grandmother' role:

+ on a domestic/practical level?
+ expectations of life?

Questions to help discussion

What choices have you made about becoming a mother to this child?

+ Was the pregnancy planned?
+ Was it a joint decision with the father?
+ Why now?

What kind of a mother would you like to be?

+ Any role models?
+ What expectations are there?
+ Are these expectations realistic?

How can you incorporate this role into the rest of your life?

+ What about the other roles you play, e.g. partner, daughter, and so on?
+ How can you juggle?
+ What do you gain?
+ What do you lose?

If you intend to return to work

+ How will you manage the work– family– life balance?
+ What needs to be in place to enable you to fulfil all these roles?

If you are not returning to work

+ How will your life change?
+ Any issues around loss of financial independence?
+ How do you imagine life will be?

How will you cope with the emotional as well as physical demands?
+ What support do you have?
+ What kind of support network do you need?
+ How much 'me-time' do you need?

Impossible expectations

As the discussion progresses, the enormity of the task ahead becomes clearer and can feel very daunting. It is vital to keep expectations realistic and not to collude with the new mother's need to be perfect. Following the brainstorm, the facilitator can suggest to the group the *impossibility* of fulfilling all these roles, skills and qualities all of the time, and introduce the need for each woman to take care of herself.

In most households, women are the lynchpin of the family and all too often put everyone else's needs before their own. For the mother to keep herself well and healthy – physically and emotionally – it is important that she looks after herself: the assumption that this is selfish or indulgent can be challenged and explored in the group.

> Women who are happy and fulfilled in themselves make better mothers and are likely to bring up healthy happy children.

Brainstorm ways to look after yourself, if necessary giving some of the following ideas to get the group started:
+ A cup of coffee and feet up when the baby is asleep.
+ A bubble bath or use essential oils in the water.
+ Sleep when the baby sleeps, even if it is 10.30 a.m.
+ Keep in touch with friends and family.
+ Accept all offers of help.
+ Any pampering/beauty treatment.
+ Massage.
+ A quiet house while someone else takes the baby for a walk.
+ Half an hour on your own reading a magazine in a coffee shop.
+ A bunch of flowers to brighten up the day.
+ Get out every day for a walk with the pram.

Feedback and ending

Summarise the main points at the end of the session and, again, emphasise that there are times when choices and compromises have to be made, as it is impossible to do everything.

Give the group the following thoughts to take away.

> It is important to look after yourself so that you can deal with the many demands placed on you. How are you doing this? How are you integrating this role into the rest of your life?

Remind the group of the next week's topic – changes in relationships. Ask the group to reflect on all current relationships and any changes they have noticed since the birth of the baby.

Equipment checklist

+ Whiteboard/flipchart and pens
+ Baby box (emergency supplies of nappies, wipes)
+ Baby mats
+ Refreshments
+ Tissues
+ Bowl to collect subs

Group case study 2
Facilitator's preparations

It is always interesting at the second session to see if everyone comes back. Sometimes we lose people along the way and often have no way of knowing why. They all seemed to enjoy last week, so I hope they will all return.

It's also tricky to know exactly what time of day to run these groups. I have tried morning and afternoons but, whatever the start time, it's hard for new mums to arrive anywhere on time. If they have other children, they sometimes have to leave early to collect them from nursery or school.

The session

Group process	Comments
Ten minutes before the group is due to start, a new member arrives and introduces herself to the facilitator and asks to join. Ros has just moved into the area and has just been told about the group by the health visitor. She is keen to meet other mums.	It is not always possible for everyone to attend the first session. When someone joins late, it may initially unsettle the group (from the third session, it becomes much more difficult to integrate a new member).
	Edith is happy for Ros to join and explains boundaries, especially the confidentiality agreement.
Check-in	
Jane (Josh), Helen (Jack), Karen (Sam and Beth), Sonita (Meenu), Jo (Esther), Milka (Janka), Natasha (Simone), Jenny (Lily), Caro (Danny), Emma (Amy) and Ros (Harry) attend.	Facilitator introduces Ros to the group.
Ros explains she has only just heard about the group. Her baby, Harry, is five months old, and she has recently moved back into the area to be nearer her parents. The other women are friendly to Ros and the rest of the check-in round proceeds.	

Group process	Comments
Helen: 'I was feeding from midnight to 4 o'clock.'	The check-in provides everyone with a chance to speak and to say how they are feeling today, and if any major events have happened in the week that they would like to share.
Karen: I counted up; I had three hours 25 minutes sleep in total last night.	
Sonita: 'This morning my husband said to me how well he had slept and did she go through the night as he hadn't heard anything – I nearly hit him!'	
Milka: 'Janka slept really well until about three weeks ago, but I think she is teething now and her sleep is all over the place.'	Sleep, or lack of it, dominates the check-in this week.
Jo: 'I've hidden the clock. I don't want to know what time it is when I'm up in the night.'	
Jane: I was up at 1 a.m., 3 a.m. and 5 a.m., then I had to waken him at 9 a.m. to get out in time.'	
Natasha: I'm really pleased that Simone has started to go through the night.'	Natasha bravely admits her sleep pattern has improved – the rest of the group are envious.
Jenny: Lily has been sleeping through since she was 10 weeks. Matthew is my problem – he keeps having nightmares.'	It's not always the babies who create sleep problems; older children can still be having disturbed sleep patterns.
Emma: 'This one is a devil at night. All I can say is, if the others had been like her, I might have just had one.'	
There is a general sharing of the trials of broken nights. Karen begins to offer solutions 'have you tried . . .?'	Facilitator re-focuses group on to how individuals are feeling and away from solutions, reminding the group it is about them, rather than the babies.
Jane describes an incident last evening with her partner. He arrived home from work, feeling very stressed and immediately said he was going out for a run as he had had a really bad day. He returned an hour later, but was quiet all evening. Jane tried to speak about this in a light-hearted way, but it was clear that she was still feeling upset.	Jane's story produces a torrent of 'men don't understand' tales and advice on what she could do. After a few moments, the facilitator intervenes – 'Jane, how are you feeling right now?' – whereupon Jane becomes tearful and describes how letdown she had felt. Facilitator allows Jane space to express her feelings of anger and frustration.

Main topic

Good response to brainstorm of roles, etc; whiteboard was quickly covered. Lots of discussion about juggling time and demands of others.

Helen is surprised at how much time the baby takes up in the day. She cannot imagine how she would cope with another and is in awe of others with more than one child: 'I'd hoped to be doing some work at home by now but, whenever I get the odd half hour to myself, I'm too exhausted to think straight and just want to collapse with a cup of coffee.'

Jo doesn't say anything but nods in agreement.

Group process	Comments
Sonita and Caro both remember those feelings first time around, and how the first six months passed in a blur.	Women with more than one child are able to give insights into future as well as current demands.
Sonita describes how exhausted she became at trying to keep on top of everything, despite help from her mother and mother-in-law, and how anxious she felt all the time. She now feels much more confident as a mother and is now wondering about going back to work – she went back full-time after her first child, but now feels she is enjoying this baby so much more that she would like to stay at home. First time around it felt like a relief to get back to normality of work, but now she would love to be at home.	They are also often more comfortable talking about negative feelings. Work issues are often a cause for concern and discussion
Jane agrees that it is much better for the child to be looked after by the mother, rather than relying on childcare. 'My mum didn't work and was always there for me, and I want to do the same for my child.'	The facilitator ensures everyone's view is aired, while remaining neutral and emphasising there is no 'right' way.
Karen agrees, but Helen has firm plans to get back to her career as soon as possible. She is ambitious and wants to return to work when Jack is five months old – he has a place at nursery and will be going there one day a week from three months old to get used to it. 'If we lived closer to our families, Jack would see lots of different people. I want him to be able to mix easily and he needs to see lots of other adults and children, so a nursery environment will be great for him socially and educationally.'	Inevitably conflicting views will emerge and the facilitator needs to contain and acknowledge them. Work can be a sensitive issue and it is important that no one feels judged for the decision they make.
Natasha explains she had no choice but to work when her sons were born and has worked full-time until recently. She has now re-married and is looking forward to staying at home with Simone, although is already wondering how she will deal with it. She has always been independent, as her first marriage ended when the boys were five and seven. She is wondering how it will feel not to be earning her own income and having to rely on her husband.	Natasha's point of view highlights the complexity of these issues. Money issues can create tension within the relationship.
Ros says she has no option but to return to work in a couple of months time: 'If I can get my brain to work again!' But she is surprised that she is now considering part-time rather than full-time as she enjoys Harry so much, even though she is exhausted all the time. 'I look at my work clothes in the wardrobe and wonder who they belong to. I can't seem to connect with that other person.'	This is the first time Ros has contributed.
This generates some hilarity and agreement as to the unexpected hazards of early motherhood.	
Milka comments she is shocked at how soon mothers have to return to work in the UK – in Slovakia most mothers stay at home and maternity leave lasts for three years!	This information from Milka causes some envy, and initiates discussion about the value placed on motherhood in our society.

Group process	Comments
With this baby, Caro feels more 'laid back' and has let go of some of the pressures she now realises she put on herself. She has changed in many ways since she has become a mother and learnt a lot about herself.	Caro picks up on Sonita's earlier theme.
Jenny's partner works away all week and comes home Friday afternoons – she sometimes finds weekends more difficult, as she is trying to fit in with him as well and her weekday routine is disrupted.	The first-time mums look rather shocked at Jenny's view.
Emma feels her life is in a constant state of chaos. Her husband works shifts, so no two weeks are the same. Her other two children often wake in the night as well as the baby. She has no nearby family support, and feels exhausted and overwhelmed all the time.	There is much empathy for Emma's situation, although again the facilitator has to steer the group away from problem-solving mode. Emma tries to put on a brave face, but looks on the brink of tears.
Emma suddenly realises the time and has to leave early to collect her son from pre-school. She leaves soon after her outpouring.	The group seems quite flat when Emma departs. Facilitator comments on this.
Ros comments that she hadn't realised it would all be so demanding.	
Natasha agrees and says she had completely forgotten just how much time a baby takes up.	The reality of motherhood is becoming apparent.
Ros asks the second-time mums when it gets easier, and both Sonita and Caro reply that, although it is always changing, it becomes different though not necessarily easier. Jenny adds that sometimes it gets worse before it gets better! Ros looks rather disappointed.	
General agreement.	
Feedback	
Natasha, Jane and Jenny say they found the discussion helpful and how good it was to put into words how they were feeling. Again, Jo doesn't speak but nods.	Facilitator draws discussion to a close and reminds group that next week is half-term so no meeting as agreed.
	Topic for the week after is changes in relationships, and facilitator suggests women could also broach this subject with their partners.

The first two sessions lay the foundations for future, more personal discussions. The aim by the end of the second session is for the group to feel settled and able to speak freely, even if individual views differ.

Facilitator's reflections

+ The group seemed to accept Ros, and she seemed happy to contribute – not always easy to join a group that is already established.
+ Noticed Ros, Sonita and Jo set off up the High Street together afterwards.

+ Sleep, or lack of it, produced lots of strong feeling – several of them are hitting the time when combination of disturbed nights and colic collide.

+ Emma doesn't seem to call Amy by name – only 'the baby'. Has a lot on her plate. Wonder how she managed with her other two. It's a shame she had to leave 10 minutes early – hope she won't have to do that every week.

+ Jane was very upset with partner – she has high ideals and standards for herself – wonder if she imposes them on Steve also? But good she was able to express how she felt. She's a bit of an earth-mother type, and she also has quite fixed ideas. I can forsee some conflict when everyone feels more settled.

+ Good mix of first-, second- and third-timers. Important for the first-timers to hear how the more experienced cope this time: a maturing into motherhood?, becoming more realistic?, or just too exhausted to worry about less important issues?!

+ Work was a dominant theme and took up much of the discussion. Helen's views came across very strongly – she was surprisingly dogmatic and seems to be used to having life organised. Her views may be intimidating to some of the others who are quieter. I found myself feeling rather irritated with her – wonder what's that about. Will have to think a bit more about that. She certainly seems to have life sorted!

+ Also ambivalence about work from some of the others. With the first baby, Sonita saw her return to work almost as a refuge, but this time she is enjoying the baby so much more. She has very strong family support, but with traditional values – her mother has never worked outside the home – I wonder was she breaking the mould by working full-time after her first baby? Maybe she wanted to be different from the previous generation?

+ Karen is determined to come up with solutions to everyone's problems – it seems hard for her to hear of anyone else's struggle – I wonder what her struggle is? When Emma was pouring her heart out, Karen got up to change Beth's nappy. I'm sure she would be much happier if we kept the focus on the babies rather than the mums – I wonder why she finds it so difficult. I've met women like Karen before: they seem to have all the answers and yet so often lack confidence beneath that bright veneer.

+ Jo still very quiet, but I feel she is very engaged with the group nevertheless – she made a definite point of talking to Ros at the end.

+ Felt we ended on a rather flat, downbeat note – hope they won't feel discouraged. I think several of them have reached the dip, when its really hard and they feel they aren't up to the job. It seems they have to reach a really low point before they can begin to accept the changes and move forward. Although they are mostly thrilled with their babies, they had not anticipated their feelings of loss of their 'old' lifestyle. It's so like the grieving process, with all the different stages, and yet grief is not something we associate with new life. I wonder if couples can prepare or whether it is an inevitable stage through which they have to go?

+ Their personalities are now beginning to emerge. It is a large group, and it can be difficult to hold all the details in my head – names, of babies, partners and some sense of their personal circumstances – but I'm beginning to get there.
+ Have sent a note to Emma to remind her we are not meeting next week as it's half-term.
+ Must remember to update contact list to include Ros.

Supporting notes
Myths of perfection

Every mother wants to do her best for her child. Of course, we all hope to have perfect children – beautiful, well-behaved, sensitive, bright, caring, kind, the list goes on. These are all elements that contribute to the picture of the 'imaginary' or 'fantasy' baby, which can emerge in the second trimester of pregnancy. And, naturally, the majority of mothers believe their new baby is beautiful and to her, he is.

Women can be critical and competitive. How many expectant mothers cringe with disapproval in the supermarket as they witness a scuffle between mother and toddler that either results in bribery or temper – from the mother or child.

'My child will never behave that way.' 'How can she give in to that tantrum?' 'She's creating a rod for her own back.' It is easy to judge and think, 'I could do it so much better.'

The perfect family unit is another unattainable myth. If the mother has a discordant family background, her desire is to get it 'right' this time, to right the wrongs of the past, will be even greater.

Aiming for perfection is a sure route to failure.

Perfection is impossible to achieve all of the time, or even some of the time. It is impossible to fulfil and accomplish the brainstorm list of roles skills and qualities. Perfection, success, failure are all harsh judgements that women impose on themselves and make life much more difficult than it need be.

Inevitably, there are times when every parent 'gets it wrong'. This can be a valuable learning opportunity for children to learn about actions and consequences, and what we can do when things go awry. It can be very important for older children to realise their parents do make mistakes sometimes, and these mistakes can often be rectified. The child then learns he does not have to be perfect either.

The process of adjustment

The early weeks of motherhood often pass in a blur. The mother may still be physically recovering from the birth, and be in some continuing discomfort. The needs and demands of the baby are all consuming: a baby cannot survive on his own and relies on others to keep him alive. The mother is this person most of the time. Issues around feeding and sleep are major concerns at this time and can induce huge anxiety for the mother.

+ To breast-feed or bottle-feed?

+ I want to breast-feed but I am having difficulty / don't like it. How long do I persevere?
+ I much prefer bottle-feeding, but feel guilty that I am not giving my child the best start in life.
+ Am I feeding too much / too little?
+ I long for the baby to sleep. Am I a bad mother?
+ I am at the end of my tether with exhaustion.
+ How long should I allow him to sleep?
+ Is he sleeping too much / too little?

These anxieties can take over and leave the new mother exhausted and with little time or energy to think about anything else. Winnicott describes this 'primary maternal preoccupation' as a unique state of mind that develops during the final stage of pregnancy and continues in the few months after birth when the mother 'loses herself to the baby to the exclusion of the outside world'.[1] Stern believes that a mother is not born 'in one dramatic defining moment' but 'gradually emerges from the cumulative work of the many months that precede and follow the actual birth'.[2] Adjustment takes place over a period of months through different stages.

0–6 weeks
+ Everything is new.
+ Lots of excitement about the baby.
+ Lots of attention from family and friends.
+ Recovery from the birth.
+ Help at home: partner may take some time off work, parents and or in-laws may be attentive and offer practical help.
+ Becoming familiar with feeding routines.
+ Expectation of disturbed nights and adjustment to feeling tired much of the time.
+ Getting to know the new baby – his likes, preferences, getting used to handling him, dressing, bathing, nappy changing, and so on.
+ First smile – around six weeks is a major milestone. This is often the first sign of the baby 'giving something back'. Up until now it can feel like a one way process.
+ A time when women are more 'home-based' than usual.

7–16 weeks
+ Breast-feeding or bottle-feeding usually more or less established.
+ Mother growing more confident about handling her baby.
+ Baby increasingly sociable and communicative as he gurgles and responds to mum's play.

But
+ Mother suffering from a build-up of exhaustion due to cumulative effects of broken nights.

+ Baby still takes up most of the mother's energy.
+ Colic may be causing mum and baby distress, especially in the evening when both are tired anyway. The magic 12-week milestone looms when colic is supposed to disappear: a great disappointment when is passes without event and the mother is still pacing the floor night after night unable to comfort her baby.
+ Feelings of loneliness may set in and the mother may be ready to get out to meet others: but where to go if all your friends work/you are new to the area/you haven't got transport and cannot face the bus?
+ Responsibility involved in being a mother is fully realised – the total commitment required.

17 weeks–6 months
+ Gradual settling down into some routine, or adjusting to no routine!
+ Baby's sleep pattern may begin to settle, so the mother is less tired.
+ Mother becomes more accustomed to her new role.
+ As her brain clears, the mother can once again think about other aspects of her life: she has more time for her partner, family, friends, work.
+ The baby becomes a part of her life – a very important part, undoubtedly – but other aspects can now also be re-integrated.

Women are most vulnerable and in need of support in the middle phase of this transition, and this is when a supportive group can be most helpful. By now, partners have returned to work and the initial flurry of visits from grandparents, family and friends may have tailed off. The reality of this new situation begins to sink in, and women often feel isolated and lonely. It is also a time when professional support is usually reduced: if the mother seems to be coping, she will be left largely to get on unless she seeks help herself.

Most episodes of depression arising in the first-year postpartum are evident between six and 12 weeks.[3] The baby's responsiveness is increasing, and a disruption to this process may have far-reaching effects on the child: several studies indicate that the quality of these early interactions is predictive of cognitive functioning at the end of the first year.[4] Every support must be given at this vulnerable time.

Daniel Stern charts the progress of Joey at six weeks, four-and-a-half months, 12 months, 20 months and four years. Drawing on facts based on extensive research, speculation based on those facts and his own imagination, Stern imagines a diary about Joey's inner life – his thoughts and feelings. At each stage, he describes Joey's new abilities, how he reacts to the world and the interplay with his parents. Even by six weeks it seems likely that the quality of the relationship built between Joey and his mother will 'act as a prototype for what he will expect to happen with other loved persons whom he encounters in life'.[5]

Andrews also demonstrates how the relationship between the baby and his parents develops. Babies at various stages during the first months have been photographed to provide a striking visual account of how these early interactions can affect the

baby, and further emphasises the need to optimise this experience for both mother and baby.[6]

Recurring themes

Realisation of what it means to be a mother

As the brainstorm indicates, the roles, skills and qualities of a mother are many and varied, and stretch way beyond babyhood. A group of mothers with children of differing ages highlights the challenges to be met at each stage, and acknowledges the responsibility, which will change as the child grows, but which never entirely disappears. To the first-time mother with a baby of seven or eight weeks, this can feel like a truly daunting task, and she may begin to feel discouraged by the enormity of it all. New mothers need lots of nurturing and encouragement themselves to build their confidence and self-esteem in this new role.

Being a mother is different from being a father

Mothers are programmed to react to their babies: a breast-feeding mother's body will prepare to produce milk on hearing her baby's cry. Mothers will sleep more lightly to ensure the baby's cry does not go unheard. A mother can soothe her own baby more effectively than anyone else. A newborn will turn his head when he hears his mother's voice. In the early weeks, it is the mother who fulfils most of the baby's needs. This can be a shock to the couple who planned to share the parenting role. Frequently, the mother will spend more time with the baby and so become more adept at handing and responding to the baby, which can leave some fathers feeling inept.

Dad is adjusting too

If support for mothers is limited, support for fathers is almost non-existent. The first-time father is all too often forgotten once initial celebrations of 'wetting the baby's head' are over. His return to work may be dreaded or envied by his partner. He may struggle to keep up with work on reduced sleep and may wish to play an active role as much as he is able. It may be difficult for him to 'get it right', while overtime or late business meetings may become more alluring than the nightly battle with colic.

The responsibility of his new role and the financial implications may weigh heavily, and there may be no one with whom he can share his worries. His partner – previously a support, friend and lover – has changed, with all her attention now being lavished on the baby. He may feel anxious and unsure about how best to handle the baby and how to support his partner at this vulnerable time. If these issues are not acknowledged between the couple, there is potential for more serious and far-reaching problems to develop.

It's OK to be 'selfish'

Being selfish is generally frowned upon, and has connotations of being self-centred, egotistical and uncaring of other people's needs and feelings. The demands placed on a mother are huge and she needs to learn to look after herself in the process. The woman determined to be 'selfless' and so be the only one to be able to meet her

child's needs, will soon find herself 'running on empty'. This can ultimately lead to self-imposed martyrdom and resentment. A mother who can take time out for herself is likely to be a happier person and, therefore, a better mother. Being able to accept help from others, and asking for it when needed, encourages a healthier dynamic in the family.

Fitting this new role into the rest of life

Although motherhood is initially all-consuming, this role is only one of the many a woman plays. She is still a partner, daughter, sister, friend, workmate, and any number of other roles she has taken on in her life. The new mother may experience conflict between the overwhelming demands of motherhood and her wish to do her absolute best for her baby, and a yearning to get 'back to normal life'. During the first months a gradual dawning may occur as she realises 'getting back' to before is not possible, and a new way forward has to be forged to include a new family member who, although tiny, impacts on every aspect of life. This is a gradual adjustment, which couples have to negotiate together in order to discover what will work for them.

Work issues

When the new mother begins to re-integrate into life outside the home, the immediate needs of the baby and the 'motherhood mindset' recedes, and thoughts of work often surface. Issues about work will have been considered during pregnancy, and have to be reviewed after the birth. Indeed, the date to return to work may be looming and preparations about childcare, working hours, and so on, need to be finalised. For some women there is no debate – the woman's income may be a crucial contribution to the family finances or she may be the major or sole earner. For women on a career path the thought of not returning to work may never have been considered.

However, returning to work can present the new mother with an unexpected and painful emotional wrench, with which she has to come to terms. Stern fully acknowledges 'the heartache of the decision' and highlights the different feelings that may emerge, depending on whether it is the woman's choice to return to work or a necessity.[7] She may experience a deep sense of loss if she has to return earlier than she is ready, and then have to contend with guilt and anger.

Strangely, the choice to stay at home full-time can also induce guilt. Some women may have to face envy from others in a less-secure financial position, friends and colleagues may be critical of the decision to give up or put on hold a career, and the loss of financial independence may present unexpected issues of responsibility and power within the relationship as the father becomes the sole earner within the family.

Decisions around work produce much anxiety and emotional turmoil, and there is no 'right' answer. But the group can provide a neutral space to think through and explore all aspects of this important area.

> No matter how much careful planning occurred before the birth, women cannot anticipate how they will feel after the birth.

For many women, the feelings they have towards their child are the strongest and most primitive feelings they have ever experienced.

The emotional aspect of mothering is often least anticipated and most challenging.

References

1 Winnicott DW. *Home is Where We Start from*. London: Penguin Books; 1986

2 Stern DN, Brushweiler N, Freeland A. *The Birth of a Mother*. London: Bloomsbury; 1998.

3 Murray L, Cooper PJ, editors. *Postpartum Depression and Child Development*. New York: Guildford; 1997.

4 Hay Dale F. Postpartum depression and cognitive development. In: Murray L and Cooper P J. *Postpartum Depression and Child Development*. New York: Guildford Press; 1997. pp. 85–110.

5 Stern DN. *Diary of a Baby*. New York: Basic Books; 1990.

6 Murray L, Andrews A. *The Social Baby*. Richmond: CP Publishing; 2000.

7 Stern DN, *et al*., op. cit.

CHAPTER 7

Session 3: Changes in relationships

The session
Aim
To personalise discussions by exploring how relationships have changed since the birth of the baby.

Objectives
+ To explore how relationships with others have changed since the birth.
+ To explore how the birth has changed the relationship the woman has with herself.

Check-in
+ How are you feeling today?
+ How has your week been?
+ How did you feel about coming today?
+ Did last week's discussion provoke any further thoughts or feelings?

Main topic
Having a baby changes everything and relationships are one area that inevitably changes when a new person joins the family. Many changes are positive, but some relationships suffer in the early weeks and months when the mother is adjusting to the many new demands made on her.

This session begins with the assumption that relationships **do** change – positively and negatively – and gives time for women to explore the changes and how they are reacting to them. Space is also given for women to discuss how they now feel about themselves, both physically and emotionally.

> **BRAINSTORM THE FOLLOWING QUESTION:** Which relationship has changed most since the birth of your baby?

partner	other children in the family	parents	in-laws
siblings	friends	work colleagues	with self

BOX 7.1 Relationships

Answers will vary, but try to allow opportunity for all the above relationships to be considered.

Questions to help discussion
In what ways have these relationships changed?
+ What are the gains/positive aspects of these changes?
+ What are the losses/negative aspects of these changes?
+ How do you feel about these changes?

How can these changes be managed?
+ What support do you need to facilitate change?
+ Are you treated any differently now that you have a/another child?

What changes have you noticed in yourself?
+ Physical changes to your body?
+ Emotional changes?
+ Any change in values?
+ Any change in attitude, e.g. to work, money issues, loss of independence?
+ Has your view of the world changed?

What is important for you now?
+ Encourage the group to think about their individual process of change.
+ Suggest that change will continue to happen as both parent and baby grow and develop.

Discuss with the group that change is normal, and that it brings up both positive and negative responses, thoughts, feelings and behaviours. This may be a new concept for individuals to accept, especially for those who tend to see life in black and white terms. Accepting and integrating the shades of grey, which ambivalence creates, is a gradual process.

Feedback and ending
Bring session to an end with a summary of the main issues discussed.
Give the group the following thoughts to take away.

Do you need to continue to think any of today's issues, or do you need to discuss them with someone else?
Can you think of any other relationships that have changed, and that we did not have time to explore?

Ask for feedback on this session and remind the group of next week's topic – parenting styles. As preparation, the group may like to think about their own childhood and talk to their partner about his memories.

Equipment checklist
+ Whiteboard/flipchart and pens
+ Baby box (emergency supplies of nappies, wipes)
+ Baby mats
+ Refreshments
+ Tissues
+ Bowl to collect subs

Group case study 3
Facilitator's preparations
It's been two weeks since we last met, as it was half-term last week, and I wonder what effect the break might have on the group. It is always a dilemma to know whether or not to continue regardless of school holidays, but it also depends on the make-up of the group – as this group has several women with other children, it seemed sensible not to meet. Had the group been mostly first-time mums it wouldn't have been an issue.

The session

Group process	Comments
Jane (Josh), Helen (Jack), Karen (Sam and Beth), Sonita (Meenu), Jo (Esther), Milka (Janka), Natasha (Simone), Jenny (Lily), Caro (Danny) and Ros (Harry) attend.	Facilitator passes on the message to the group and distributes the contact list.
Emma sends a message that she will be unable to attend today as her middle child is unwell.	
Check-in	
Jane expresses concern for Emma as she thought she was upset when she left the group last time. Jane saw Emma at the supermarket during the week, but Emma was unable to chat as she had all three children with her and Amy was fractious.	Facilitator suggests she will drop Emma a note on behalf of the group to wish her well and hope she is able to attend next week.
Natasha really missed the group last week – she is surprised that she is enjoying it so much as she was worried before she came along that she would feel like an 'old' mum and have nothing in common with others. In fact, it gives her time to think about how she is with this new baby.	Two week gap since last meeting owing to school holidays.
Sonita agrees that the group provides a focal point to the week.	

Group process	Comments
Karen's husband is a teacher and had last week off school for half-term, which was a great help to Karen as he was around to help out with the twins, and they could have a baby each when they went out. Karen enjoyed one-to-one time with each baby, rather than always having to divide her time between the two of them. She has found it hard this week to be on her own again, and has also been looking forward to meeting this week.	Until now Karen has played 'joker' in the group, but this week she is more serious and comes across as more 'real' in that she is admitting that life can be stressful. The check-in continues with space for everyone to contribute.
Jenny is last to check-in and she has been thoughtfully listening to everyone else. She speaks very quietly and tells the group that she had a stillborn daughter, Cecily, 18 months before her son was born and she would have been six last week. 'This is always a difficult time of year for me and it doesn't seem to be getting any easier. This year, now that I have another girl, it seems even harder. I keep wondering what Cecily would be like now. Matthew knows he had a big sister who died and I want Lily to know as well – she is still part of the family and we must never forget her.'	The group listens attentively to Jenny's story. She becomes distressed as she speaks but carries on slowly. Jenny's story has a profound effect on the group, with many of the women close to tears.
Sonita responds: 'I'm lucky enough to have a six-year-old daughter, but I can empathise with you, Jenny, as I had a late miscarriage four years ago and still find myself thinking of what might have been.'	Jenny's disclosure enables other women in the group to talk about past sadness and grief in an open and supported way.
Jane adds that she had had fertility treatment for several years and Josh was conceived on their third IVF attempt. They were about to give up, and had years of highs and lows, and she had almost given up hope of ever having a child.	The facilitator allows the check-in to extend beyond the usual time to ensure everyone can participate in this important discussion as issues around loss are explored.
Main topic	
Most of the group feel the that it is the relationship with their partner that has changed most since the birth, and this discussion takes up most of the session.	'Which relationship has changed most for you since the birth of this child?'
Sonita describes how different it is for her this time around. Her husband, Raj, has just changed his job. He now has a longer journey to work and more responsibility, which means he is rarely home before 9 p.m. Sonita is finding this a great strain, as he had been very hands-on with their first child, Asha. 'When he does finally get home, Asha is in bed but really misses seeing daddy in the week. I am usually pacing the floor with Meenu, and I can barely speak two words to him I'm so exhausted. I know he's finding this new job really tough, but I have nothing left to give him at the end of the day.'	

Group process	Comments
Emma and Caro agree, but Natasha describes a very different scenario: 'Martin doesn't want to miss out on Simone the way he did with his children from his first marriage – he worked all hours and that was part of the reason for his divorce. This time he's around a lot, can't do enough for Simone, which is lovely but . . . I feel like I'm invisible. He's the one who leaps out of bed as soon as Simone stirs. We were so close when I was pregnant, now he hardly touches me.'	Group interacting naturally without any input from the facilitator. Natasha is missing the intimacy attained in pregnancy.
Caro: 'I wish Martin could speak to Matt. He hasn't quite grasped that we now have two children and its not double the work – it's ten times as much. Tom was sleeping through at nine weeks and our sex life was back on track by this stage. Danny is now 14 weeks and shows no sign of going through. I can't imagine ever wanting sex again!'	
Jo: 'I miss it just being us . . . I love Esther to bits but I do miss how peaceful it used to be when it was just the two of us.'	Jo is finally relaxed enough to contribute to the discussion.
General discussion about sex – too much or too little – which highlights the diversity of feelings and underlines there is no 'normal'.	The group's ease in discussing an intimate subject is a measure of its cohesion and security. Everyone joins in to some extent apart from Ros, who looks rather uncomfortable.
Discussion develops into further exploration of the loss on intimacy between the couple. First-time mums, and Jane in particular, can be nervous of how their partner handles the baby. Jane knows she shouldn't keep on telling him how to do it, but cannot help herself. This is creating some tension between them, which last night ended in a row.	It also takes time for the father to adjust to his new role and to learn how to handle the baby.
Jenny's partner works away all week and is at home weekends, so she is constantly having to get used to something different, making weekends fraught. 'All week I know it's all down to me, and then at the weekend I expect Rob to help with Lily, but he finds Matthew much easier to cope with.'	In families with more than one child, the father often looks after the older child(ren), while the mother focuses on the baby.
Caro also reflects on how her partner changed during the first year or so of Tom's life as he gradually grew into his new role. 'Ben eventually realised he couldn't play football every Saturday afternoon, and train twice a week, and go to the pub on a Friday after work, but it took him until Tom was about a year and lots of rows along the way!'	
Milka feels she has become more dependent on Phil since Janka arrived. 'She has brought us closer together, but now I also miss my family more.'	Several of the group have families who live some distance away.

Group process	Comments
	Facilitator is aware that Ros has lost interest in the discussion and has begun to play with Harry and Jenny's daughter, Lily who is sitting next to her. Facilitator invites her to join in the discussion: 'Ros, do you think your relationship has changed at all?'
Ros laughs and replies: 'You could say that. Harry's father left when I was eight months' pregnant. He went back to his wife. My relationship has changed all right – I don't have one any more! I feel a bit of a freak here. You all seem so happy and settled and I'm back living with my parents – at 33, for heavens sake.' Ros laughs mirthlessly, but tears immediately start rolling down her face. Jenny who is sitting next to her puts a hand on her arm as Ros pours out her story. Pete had separated from his wife shortly before they got together. Ros's pregnancy wasn't planned, but Pete seemed happy about it after a while – his wife hadn't wanted children. However, as the pregnancy progressed Ros sensed that he was distancing himself from her and was no longer involved in making plans for the baby. He left her just as she was going on to maternity leave.	The group digest this information and make noises of support for Ros. The facilitator observes that Ros sounds angry as well as upset.
Ros explains her emotions swing from fury to despair, but often she is too tired to feel anything. 'I'm glad you all know now. I wasn't sure I would be able to tell you. I wanted to come to meet other normal women – and to get out of the house – my mum is driving me round the bend with her advice, which is 30 years out of date.'	The facilitator thanks Ros for her honesty and, after some further discussion, Ros says she is feeling better now and could we move on. Mood of the group lightens again.
Discussion now naturally moves on to focus on how relationships have changed with their own mothers.	
Both Helen and Jane say their relationship with their mothers is even better now – both are very supportive. Jane's mum lives nearby and is already an important part of Josh's life. Helen's mother is also a great support but, owing to distance, this is mainly over the telephone. 'My two older sisters live near my parents and they have five children between them. They have the support of the whole extended family, which I didn't like so much when I was younger but I can appreciate now.' Helen goes on to explain that much of the family's social life at 'home' revolves around the synagogue. Moving away was greeted with dismay by both sets of parents, and there is pressure to move closer to home.	

Group process	Comments
Sonita takes up the theme: 'I think I appreciate my mum more since Meenu arrived. I was the eldest of five children, and my mum always seemed to be immersed in babies and never worked outside the home when I was growing up. I wanted to be different, so when I had Asha, I was determined to juggle work and family. It's only now I realise what my mum did for all of us . . . oh, I think that's the first time I've admitted that even to myself.'	Sonita needs a few moments to fully digest what she has just said and is clearly emotional. She has obviously struck a chord with Milka, also.
Milka: 'In the few months since Janka was born I have missed my mum more than in the past 10 years. I also feel guilty that I am so far away – my mum dotes on her other grandchildren But I know she will never be able to have quite the same relationship with Janka – they'll both miss out.'	The role of grandparents is explored and the value of this unique relationship discussed.
Natasha's mother is very different now from when Natasha had her first child 12 years ago – Natasha can see she has aged a lot in that time: her arthritis has deteriorated and she doesn't feel confident in handling Simone. Natasha feels guilty, as she feels her mother needs her to spend more time with her, and yet Natasha has her hands full with her own life.	Natasha's story illustrates how life is ever-changing, and how the balance changes as our own parents age and become more dependent.
Caro: 'I feel guilty, too, but about my mother-in-law. My mum died of breast cancer when I was pregnant with Tom (now three years), so my mum will never know my children. I really miss her. I could do with her help right now. I'm worried about my dad. Although he loves the boys, I know he's lonely. My mother-in-law is great – she's really helpful, but I get resentful because I want my mum to be here. I know it's really unfair on her, but I can't seem to help it. I can be snappy with her when she's only trying to help.	Caro's voice falters, but she carries on.
Jane says she cannot imagine Caro being snappy with anyone, and almost dismisses what Caro has said.	Although Jane's comment to Caro was meant kindly, it denies Caro the opportunity to fully express how she is feeling. Facilitator brings focus back to Caro to give her more space to talk about her grief.
Caro: 'Sometimes I feel fine and then other days it all hits me again. She died nearly four years ago – surely I should be over it by now.'	Facilitator reassures Caro that there is no time limit to grief, and wonders if Caro is reliving the period when Tom was at this stage, and her grief has become acute again.
Caro thinks about this and agrees. 'Danny looks so like Tom. I think I have gone back to how I felt then. I looked at some old photos, and all I could think was that mum wasn't there.'	The session is now coming to a close and the facilitator asks if anyone has experienced a major change in other relationships.

Group process	Comments
Sonita is really missing the one-to-one closeness she had with her older daughter: 'Asha was an only child for so long – we were really close, especially after my miscarriage four years ago when I thought I probably wouldn't have another child. It's very different now – as I said earlier, Raj is working longer hours and I feel Asha is missing out from both of us. She's loves Meenu, but she's really grumpy with me.'	
Jenny and Natasha empathise with Sonita and discuss how their other children cope with the new arrival, and how they both struggle to meet everyone's demands – and what happens when they cannot!	
Feedback and ending	
Caro: 'Isn't it funny how many of us feel guilty, for lots of different reasons – I thought I was the only one.'	As the session draws to a close, the facilitator checks how everyone is feeling, as this has been an emotional session. She comments on the feeling of support that seems to be developing among the women. She suggests the group may like to think further about how other relationships have changed – with siblings or friends, for example.
General nodding in agreement.	
Helen: 'I'm glad I didn't have time to talk about my mother-in-law. She's coming for the weekend – no doubt with more of her special cheesecake. She says it's for me, but I think she's worried I'm not looking after her darling son well enough.'	Reminder of next week's topic – parenting styles. Group may wish to think about this topic: memories of childhood – what they enjoyed and didn't enjoy. Also discuss with partner.

Facilitator's reflections

Good session today. They are really beginning to trust each other and open up. Lots of emotion surfaced.

✦ I'm a bit surprised at so much concern for Emma – she must have made quite an impact in the first two sessions.

✦ Jenny, Ros and Caro are all having tough times – it seemed to help them to share their problems.

✦ Spoke to Ros at the end – she was quite upbeat, but her situation is difficult. The father is happy to pay maintenance but Ros doesn't want him to see Harry. Oh dear, I really wanted to say to her to be careful about making such a big decision but, of course, I couldn't. I wonder how that will work out in the future?

✦ Karen dropped the joker role today and was more able to talk about how life really is for her. So hard having twins, though she appears to cope well, or is that what she wants everyone to think? She actually seemed very upset by what Jenny said and the subsequent contributions from the rest of the group. She didn't contribute herself – I thought she stayed around a bit at the end when I

was talking to Ros – I had the impression she wanted to see me, but she had left by the time I was free.

✦ Several seem to re-evaluating the importance of family and, in particular, their relationship with their own mother. This often seems to happen: a need to establish ourselves that might mean distancing from the family and then re-connecting when children arrive – the ebb and flow of family life, I suppose. I wonder how I will cope with that stage when my boys strike out on their own?

✦ I've just realised something today – I'm quite envious of Natasha. I, too, got divorced when my boys were young and met Ian a few years later. Ian had three children from his first marriage, but I hoped we could have a child together. But Ian was adamant we couldn't afford it and, of course, he was absolutely right, but it took me quite a few years to get over the yearning. I guess I look at Natasha and those memories come back . . . need some time to think a bit more about it all.

Phone call from Karen today

Not sure she will be able to come again – felt very upset after yesterday's session when Jenny had been describing her stillbirth. Karen had had a termination when she was 21, and all the memories of that time of her life were evoked by Jenny's story. Although she knows it was the right decision for her, she has spells of being consumed by guilt and regret. Her partner does not know about it – it happened long before she met him and she has tried to block it from her mind. She was living abroad when it happened and so did not even tell her family, who are Catholic and would have been shocked. The memories were around during her early pregnancy, and she did confide in her sister, which was a relief. Since the birth, she has tried to blot them out by focusing on the twins. She did not expect to feel this way in the group and wonders if she can return.

Karen feels she might need some time to talk through her feelings around the termination. I reassured her that it was not uncommon for past issues to be rekindled and counselling may enable her to come to terms with the past. Gave Karen some options about counselling. I have a colleague who also works at the surgery. Karen could be referred by her GP, and the counselling would therefore be quite separate from the group. Also gave the number of the local counselling agency and some independent practitioners. Karen will give these options some thought and will think about continuing with the group.

Supporting notes

By session three, the group will usually have settled and become used to the format and be ready to tackle some of the more emotional topics. Changes to relationships after the birth may not have been anticipated during pregnancy, and it can take time to accept and work through.

Stern charts many of the changes in relationships relevant to all new mothers, including:[1]

✦ the shift from daughter to mother

+ turning toward other women
+ seeing husband/partner differently
+ forming new triangles with the influence of the baby's presence
+ finding a new role in the family
+ finding a new place in society.

In the early weeks, the woman is usually physically and emotionally consumed by the infant, leaving little time or energy for other relationships, and it takes time for the changes to close relationships to become apparent. Stern sees the early months as an adjustment period, when the woman makes the journey from her fantasy of motherhood to reality. However, this transition from her 'irrevocably lost past' to 'an undefined future' can be a daunting one, and can present the new vulnerable mother with challenges as well as triumphs.

Recurring themes

The assumption underlying this session is that many relationships **will** change following the birth. If the facilitator can convey the inevitability and normality of change, it helps give permission to talk through these changes. Often the changes will be positive, but it is also to be expected that some changes will be difficult or even painful. For first-time parents, the birth marks both the beginning of being a family and also the loss of being a couple. Likewise, each addition to the family marks a new era in the family history.

This session aims to give women space to explore the gains and losses that they experience with the new arrival. It is just as important to acknowledge the losses as it is to celebrate the gains.

Partner

It is often the woman's relationship with her partner, which changes most after the birth of a child. Stern suggests the relationship has to be re-invented in the light of the baby's arrival, and Raphael-Leff believes parenthood offers 'opportunities to renegotiate emotional expectations' within a relationship.[2] Yet during pregnancy these changes can be difficult to imagine or prepare for, and it is only with hindsight that many couples realise the extent of the change that has occurred within the relationship.

Involvement in the pregnancy and birth

Many expectant fathers play an active part in the pregnancy by attending antenatal classes and learning how to support their partners during the birth. A new level of closeness and intimacy can develop as the pregnancy progresses and the birth becomes imminent.

However, it can be distressing to witness their partner's pain and discomfort at the birth, and some men have to contend with the mixed emotions of joy at the delivery while feeling disturbed or even traumatised by the events preceding or following the birth.

If events have not gone to plan and there is perhaps concern for the baby, resulting in admission to the special care baby unit, the father can feel torn as to where he should be – with the baby or with his partner. In the aftermath of this busy time, it can be many months before the man has the opportunity to think about and deal with his feelings.

The early weeks

Paternity leave provides some opportunity to strengthen the bonds of the new family unit, and this can be a very special time for the family to be together. However, as the father returns to the normal routine of working life and mother and baby are left alone together, she inevitably becomes more expert at handling her baby and learning to 'read' the baby's moods and needs.

Inevitably, the father tends to be not so practised in handling the baby or picking up his signals. This can be frustrating for even the most committed father, and he can begin to feel a lack of confidence in his new role, which may lead to a sense of inadequacy and distance. These feelings can deepen as the new mother can hardly stop herself from saying: 'No, no; this way is better', 'You don't do it (changing a nappy, feeding, burping and so on) like that', 'Let me show you how to . . .'

Time demands

It is impossible for any couple to prepare themselves for the physical challenges that accompany the arrival of a baby: broken nights, the sheer amount of time the feeding/changing ritual takes – to be repeated many times a day; snatched or disturbed meals; endless washing – how many outfits can a baby get through in a day?; the list goes on. All the 'busyness' of the baby-focused activity probably means there is little time for the couple themselves, and the intimacy of the pregnancy can diminish.

Fathers trying to incorporate their new role into their working lives may struggle with the many new demands made upon them, and feel the support they previously enjoyed from their partner is now lacking as her time and attention is dominated by the baby. Traditionally, men do not share the same type of emotional support network that many women benefit from, thus increasing feelings of isolation. There may be a reluctance to acknowledge these feelings, even to themselves, and some men may cope by further distancing, which can be, at the very least, hurtful to their partner and, at worst, damaging to the relationship.

Sex

The woman will still be recovering from the birth in the early weeks and sex may be the last thing on her mind. Exhaustion and possible physical discomfort or pain are not the ideal ingredients for lovemaking. Sleep has to be grabbed whenever possible and, of course, the new mother is adjusting slowly to the fact that the total oblivion of sleep may be a forgotten pleasure as she learns to rest with one ear listening out for the baby. The all-consuming energy required by the baby uses up the mother's physical and emotional resources, leaving little for her partner. The baby must be the mother's primary focus – he is reliant on her for his survival, and all other

relationships seem to take a back seat at this stage. Sex may be one activity that she can limit in order to cope with other demands over which she has no control.

It is possible that the couple's sex life will have altered either as a result of the pregnancy or during the course of the pregnancy: sexual activity may have increased or decreased at different times during the previous months. Even if the couple is looking forward to a resumption of a 'normal' sex life after the birth, the mother's readiness to resume a physical relationship with her partner will depend on many physical and emotional factors as her body heals.

This lack of a sexual relationship can further add to the reduction of intimacy between the couple, as the father feels more excluded from the intense relationship developing between mother and child. He attempts to work out how this new role will affect him and how he fits into this new family dynamic.

Responsibility

For many new fathers, the weight of the responsibility that accompanies a child can feel overwhelming. The father may take on more financial responsibility in the family as he becomes the sole or main earner. If he is not working or providing an income, there may be increased pressure to provide as the lack of financial security causes tension within the couple. Even if the financial burden is shared between the couple, the lasting commitment to the family unit and all that that entails dawns gradually in the early months, and can be a scary prospect.

Depression

A cluster of the issues described above provide fertile conditions for depression to develop, and indeed the term 'male PND', which has come into being in recent years, provides an explanation of how many men feel after the birth.

The term PND is used in everyday speech to cover a broad spectrum of conditions, ranging from 'baby blues' to puerperal psychosis. Nevertheless, this very general phrase is understood by most people to indicate a level of distress that is difficult to manage and is specific to the postnatal period. It encompasses and acknowledges the hormonal and emotional changes that occur after birth. Likewise, male PND, even if it is not officially recognised as an illness in its own right, elicits a common understanding of psychological pain induced by the arrival of the baby.

Depression in men in the postnatal period can be easily missed simply because no one is on the lookout for it. The mother has regular contact with health professionals and, although the focus is on the baby, the perceptive health professional will also assess the mother's emotional well-being. It is unlikely that anyone will routinely enquire about the father's physical or mental health at this time.

Many men find it difficult to divulge their feelings, and may find it particularly hard to admit to emotional distress at a time when they are expected to be 'strong' and focused on their partner and baby. Even in relationships that are usually mutually supportive, the woman's attention is likely to be diverted, and she may not pick up that her partner is struggling in any way.

The new father may cope with these feelings by spending more time in his usual

comfort zone: work, the pub or sport may be safe havens at a time when home-life has been turned upside down. He may feel unsure and unclear how to develop this new role. Feelings of vulnerability and exclusion from the bond of the mother–baby attachment may mean some men will seek attention elsewhere. This is a stressful time for many couples, presenting opportunities for any previous flaws in the relationship to re-surface and cause added complications.

Other children in the family

During a second pregnancy, many women worry that they will be unable to love a second child as much as they love the first. There is an anxiety that their love will have to be shared out between subsequent children, and so the first child will receive less. In fact, each child brings with him another 'consignment' of love for the mother to bestow. Nevertheless, for some women the loss of this exclusive relationship with the firstborn can be poignant. In an attempt to assuage the guilt, the mother may overcompensate and lavish much attention on the first child to reassure him that nothing has changed. In turn, this can lead to more guilt about the lack of attention she is paying to the new baby! This vicious circle of guilt is a familiar one to many mothers, and it can take time for a woman to accept that she has enough love for both children.

Of course, second (third, fourth, and beyond) children react in differing ways to a new baby – sibling rivalry is common and often feared by loving parents. Although jealousy can be displayed directly to a new sibling, the rage can be more subtly directed towards the mother. This type of rejection only adds to the mother's guilt, and she can again find herself in the vicious circle described above. On a bad day, she can feel as if she is failing both children, which can deepen her sense of inadequacy at a vulnerable time.

When the second child is born, the firstborn's supremacy is displaced, as the second born becomes the baby of the family. When a third child is born, the firstborn has already established himself as a 'big brother', but the second, now middle child, loses his 'baby rights' to the latest edition. Middle children can be confused: neither the oldest nor the youngest, they can find it difficult to establish a particular role within the family.

Parents and in-laws
Grandparents

When new parents are 'born', relationships with the couple's own parents alter. The grandparenting role may be eagerly adopted or reluctantly accepted as the generations all move up a level. While there will be many enriching gains, there may be feelings of loss and sadness as previous alliances adjust to the new member of the family.

The new parents' own grandparents may well have played a significant role in their childhoods as families were much less mobile 20 to 30 years ago. The extended family – comprising grandparents, aunts, uncles and cousins – may have lived nearby and been in frequent contact. Even the terms 'Granny' and 'Grandad' conjure up

storybook images of retired folk with plenty of time on their hands to help out.

Nowadays, grandparents in their 50s and 60s may still be working or, if retired, may be having their own 'gap year' or living a busy life crammed with their own activities and pastimes, and be unavailable or unwilling to help out. Increased mobility in the housing and job markets may also mean family live at a considerable distance, and so are unable to provide 'hands-on' help.

Although the older generation can provide an invaluable source of support, memories of their own early parenting experience may have become rather idealised, as the past is remembered through rose-tinted glasses. Memories of how perfect their own offspring was can sometimes reinforce the new parents' lack of confidence, and be decidedly unhelpful.

The lessons learnt during their own years of parenting mean grandparents can develop a very different type of relationship with grandchildren, compared to the relationships they had with their own offspring. Whereas parents are involved with all the responsibilities and pressures of everyday life, grandparents can concentrate on the child and give time and energy and enjoy the fun bits of parenting. They may also be more financially secure, and so able to 'spoil' and indulge the grandchildren in a way that wasn't possible with their own children.

When it works well, grandparents can be an enormous support. But it can be a fine line between helpful advice and interference, and tensions can arise until everyone settles into their new roles and boundaries are clarified. The relationship between grandparent and grandchild will also be coloured and influenced by the relationships already in place between the new parents and their parents, and previous conflicts may either deepen or heal.

Mothers

The birth of a child means that a daughter has now become a mother herself and so has joined her own mother in a common role. Mother–daughter relationships are rarely consistently tranquil, and can be fraught with the polarities of harmony and discord, closeness and rejection, love and hate, as the women strive to become accustomed to their emerging roles.

There may be the chance to build closer ties and to heal old hurts as the daughter's empathy with her mother grows. On the other hand, if there is a history of abuse or abandonment, the daughter may have even less understanding of her mother's motives or action.

The mother who was adopted will have achieved something which her (adopted) mother was unable to do, which may create feelings of envy in the grandmother or reawaken the pain of her own infertility.

Mothers-in-law often receive a bad press and can be portrayed as both figures of fun and derision. Mothers and sons traditionally form a close bond that is quite different from the mother–daughter relationship: mothers will often say their sons are more affectionate and will look after their mothers in times of difficulty. The son's wife or partner may be viewed as a rival, and the birth of her child may lead to a deterioration of the relationship.

Sometimes rivalry can exist between the mother and mother-in-law as they vie for the grandchild's affections. Some sensitivity between them can ensure the new parents do not feel torn loyalties, which may lead to further tensions.

Fathers

Pregnancy, birth and the early weeks of parenting remain the province of women, so men do not feature prominently at this time. Fathers may be obliged to accept now that 'his little girl' has actually grown up, and the new mother may need to let go of her idealised view of daddy. The new father will consider his relationship with his own father, and decide whether to follow in the same mould or change it.

Absent parents

Parents can be 'absent' for a number of reasons: bereavement, divorce, work commitments, estrangement or adoption.

The death of a parent, either recently or in childhood, can be particularly painful to bear at this stage, and may re-awaken grief from the past or induce a new level of grief, which needs to be worked through. The fact that the lost parent will never see or know the new baby is hard to endure, and so the baby's arrival may be bittersweet, and means the mother is facing a wide range of emotions all at once.

Parents absent because of divorce or estrangement may also be sorely missed, although a new birth can provide an incentive to re-build broken relationships. However, having now become a parent, feelings of anger and hurt may emerge at the previous abandonment.

The adopted child who becomes a parent may have new questions about the birth parents, and a search for them may be contemplated. Ambivalent and confusing feelings about birth parents may be unexpected, especially if the relationship with the adoptive parents is good.

Intermittent absences may also have had an effect on the relationship with parents. Work commitments may mean a parent, usually the father, may have been unavailable for family life. Fathers employed abroad or in the armed services or similar may have spent periods working away from home. Some shift patterns or long working hours may have meant that even if dad was there, he saw little of the children or the children had to be quiet if he was asleep. These circumstances may influence the choice of partner or may become an issue for the new mother, if she foresees history repeating itself.

If the new father's own father was absent for any reason, and so he has not had the experience of being fathered himself, he may find his new role daunting, as he has no role model to follow.

Siblings

The birth of the next generation can ignite past sibling relationships as old rivalries and alliances are re-enacted. It may be an opportunity for an older sister or brother to initiate a younger sibling into the role of parent, and offer advice and support. Or it might provide fertile ground for competition for the best, cleverest, prettiest baby among previously rivalling siblings.

Tensions may arise if siblings start a family 'out of turn', for example, when the youngest is the first to reproduce.

Even in current times, the gender of the baby may be of significance in some families: a boy to carry on the family name can still be viewed as a positive attainment.

Having a child can mean that families re-connect, and more importance may be given to family gatherings such as christenings, birthdays, anniversaries, and so on. Siblings may also want their own children to have good relationships with their cousins, although again this will depend on the experience the siblings had in childhood.

Only children

Of course, not all new parents have siblings, and the creation of a family of their own may rekindle feelings around this absence. Reasons to have just one child can vary from an active choice to medical, social or financial reasons why more children may not have been possible or advisable. These reasons are not always explained within families, and the mystery surrounding the past can make it difficult even to ask about the circumstances.

Bernice Sorensen explores 'the shame of being an only', and her research concludes that only children experience 'a lack through not having siblings'.[3] Her website provides an opportunity for exploration, acknowledgement and validation of this experience.

It is always possible that a sibling may have died at some point beyond the surviving child's memory, or that he or she was a 'replacement' child. The raw pain of losing a child is hard to contemplate, and the way grief is handled will also depend upon the family culture, ranging from being able to talk about the child in a natural way to the whole subject being taboo and, therefore, unspoken. Only children may feel pressurised to produce grandchildren to alleviate some sadness of their parents.

The individual's experience of being an only child can also colour future choices about the number of children planned. Some people may want several children to avoid recreating their own solitary, and perhaps lonely, experience, while others may feel they benefited from their parent's exclusive attention.

Friends

Early motherhood is a time when women naturally look to other women for guidance and support. Friends who already have children may be sought out for advice, as pregnancy and birth stories are shared and feeding experiences evaluated. Stitches, cracked nipples, bowel habits of the baby all become routine topics of conversation, and all forge deeper relationships with other mothers. Friendships with women also keen to have children may deepen. However, some friendships may become strained. Women desperately wanting to conceive or who have suffered miscarriages may find it too painful to be around anyone who has been 'successful' in having a baby.

Friends who are childless by choice may find the new mother's preoccupation with her new baby irritating, and feel they have lost her. It may be difficult to accept that

she is no longer there for long chats on the telephone, or available for shopping or evenings out. These friendships may become more distant as the new mother has little time or energy for anything apart from the baby. These friendships often recover a few months later when the new mother finds some emotional space to engage again with other people, and at that point her friends without children may provide a welcome relief from the routine of childrearing.

Work colleagues

Decisions regarding a return to work will be contemplated during pregnancy and a tentative choice made. For some women, of course, there is no real choice and they will have to work for financial necessity. Some women want to have the minimum amount of time off to ensure there is little disruption to their careers. Others plan to return part-time, to retain part of their 'old' life while contributing to the family income.

Whatever plans were made during pregnancy, there is no guarantee that the women will *feel* the same after the birth. When the baby is two to three months old, and the return to work becomes more imminent, some women will be looking forward to a return to their old life, while others realise their priorities have changed and that work has a different place in their lives. The pressure to find good childcare, get the baby into a routine, hopefully sleeping through the night, as well as contemplating leaving the baby for an extended time can present many challenges.

Work colleagues may be surprised at the changes in the new mother, and she may struggle to integrate two very different aspects of her life.

The woman's relationship with herself
Emotional changes

Changes in how the mother feels about herself will become apparent only gradually as the mother matures into her newest role. She may now view the world through the eyes of a mother, rather than an autonomous individual, and the horror of life and world events, especially where children are involved, may be too awful to contemplate. Media news coverage is often avoided and news items involving abuse or neglect of children can be too distressing to tolerate, as the new mother's emotions are often close to the surface.

As her sense of responsibility sinks in, she may become increasingly aware of her own vulnerability and mortality, and question who will look after her baby if something were to happen to her. These are disturbing and yet normal thoughts that can plague the woman in the early days.

Values, attitudes and future plans may all be re-assessed in the light of parenthood, and it is to be hoped the couple can jointly deal with these issues by recognising and discussing the effects of change. However, communication can be limited in the early months when it seems impossible to be able to drink a hot cup of coffee together, never mind explore the minefield of changing feelings.

Changes to her body

Motherhood almost always leaves its mark physically, and many women never fully recover their pre-pregnancy body. Stretch marks, stitches, caesarean scars, weight gain, breasts that never regain their pertness leave many women less than happy with their bodies postnatally. These days, when slimness and perfection go hand in hand, and celebrities are feted for losing all signs of the pregnant body with the delivery of the placenta, it can be at best disheartening and at worst a real blow to self-esteem for the woman to accept these changes. She may need time to come to terms with her altered shape, and even delay a return to her sex life while this acceptance takes place.

Women with a history of eating disorders can find pregnancy challenging as well as disturbing, as they increasingly lose control of their body shape. They may find it difficult to nourish themselves adequately during pregnancy and may struggle to deal with the conflict between a loss of control of their own body and a desire to nourish the growing baby. This ambivalence can be very distressing and may continue after birth if the mother 'blames' the child for her transformed shape. The Eating Disorders Association estimate there are one-and-a-half million sufferers of eating disorders, diagnosed and undiagnosed, in the UK.[5] Even if not current sufferers, stress can re-awaken past difficulties and pregnancy may well be a trigger.

> Changes in relationships are natural after the birth; these can have positive and negative effects.
> It is important to acknowledge the losses as well as the gains that change brings.
> It is valuable to recognise the internal and emotional changes, as well as the external and practical changes.

References

1 Stern DN, Brushweiler N, Freeland A. *The Birth of a Mother.* London: Bloomsbury; 1998.

2 Raphael-Leff J. *Pregnancy: the inside story.* London: Karnac; 1993.

3 Sorensen B. Spoilt or spoiled: the shame of being an only. *Therapy Today.* 2006; **17**, 3: pp. 38–41

4 www.onlychild.org.uk (accessed 23 March 2008).

5 www.b-eat.co.uk (accessed 23 March 2008).

CHAPTER 8

Session 4: Parenting style

The session
Aim
To explore different styles of parenting.

Objectives
+ To explore and share memories of childhood within a safe environment.
+ To examine different parenting styles.
+ To discuss aspects that make-up a positive parenting approach.

Check-in
The group will now be very familiar with the check-in routine, and will need little encouragement to share how they are today and significant events from their week.
+ How are you feeling this week?
+ Is there anything left over from our discussion last week on changing relationships?

Main topic

This session can be emotional for some women and may evoke feelings that they did not anticipate. The facilitator needs to be very sensitive to the mood within the room.

BRAINSTORM THE FOLLOWING QUESTION: When you think back to your childhood what, either good or bad, comes to mind first?

Holidays	Days out	Siblings	Family meal times
Fun times	Playing with friends	School	Discipline
Christmas	Mum crying	Dad drunk	My bedroom
My dog dying	My bedroom		

BOX 8.1 Childhood

The oldest, the baby or the one in the middle?	The peacemaker or mediator?
The naughty or mischievous one?	The scapegoat or the favourite?
The 'black sheep' or the 'golden girl'?	An only child?

BOX 8.2 Position/role within the family?

Questions to help discussion

The following questions encourage the group to focus on their own family background. The first two will usually provoke spontaneous discussion, and the examples given below need be used only if the group fail to come up with ideas of their own.

What was your family 'culture'?

This question will give a more detailed view of family values. What were your family's attitudes towards:

+ gender?
+ work?
+ education?
+ money?
+ possessions?
+ appearance?
+ religion?
+ morals?

How did your family deal with:

+ problems?
+ crises?
+ celebrations?

How did your parents get on with:

+ each other?
+ their own parents?
+ the extended family?
+ friends?
+ neighbours?
+ work colleagues?
+ the local community?

Exploration of the above questions will enable the group to think about this final question. Again some examples are given, but it is more meaningful if individuals can think of their own.

What would be your family motto?
+ Just get on with it.
+ We don't tell anyone else our business.
+ Always look on the bright side.

What was your partner's experience?
It is useful to gain insight into the partner's background to introduce how conflicts may arise within the couple if opposing values have been internalised.

The second half of the session provides a forum to discuss the development of each individual's own parenting style. A brainstorming session on the range of parenting styles provides a good base for further discussion – this material would be generated from memories and information on how other families, known to each group member, function.

What different styles of parenting have you observed?
+ Nurturing.
+ Critical.
+ Encouraging.
+ Fair.
+ Blaming.
+ Positive.
+ Strict.

The discussion can now move on to consider what approach each person is most comfortable with, and how they might begin to put this into practice.

Taking your own background into account, how would you like your family unit to function?
+ What have you learnt from your parents?
+ What features will you carry on into your own family?
+ What aspects will you change to create a different experience for your children?
+ What values do you want to pass onto your children?
+ What sort of family atmosphere would you like to build?
+ How will you manage conflict within the family?
+ How will you manage any differences in attitude or approach with your partner?

Feedback and ending
The potential material generated at this session is vast and all aspects cannot possibly be covered. It must be made clear to the group that the session is intended to prompt further thoughts and deliberations, which each individual can continue with her

partner. The group is not providing a perfect parenting plan, but aims to encourage parents to think about the experience they would like their children to have. This group is not able to give the answers, merely to ask the questions!

Give the group the following thoughts to take away.

What would you like your family motto to be?

How can you and your partner make this motto work?

Ask for feedback on this session and remind the group of next week's topic – an exploration of feelings, especially difficult feelings. As preparation, the group might like to notice their own feelings, moods and reactions during the coming week.

Equipment checklist
+ Whiteboard / flipchart and pens
+ Baby box (emergency supplies of nappies, wipes)
+ Baby mats
+ Refreshments
+ Tissues
+ Bowl to collect subs

Group case study 4
Facilitator's preparations
Half-way through the group this week. Last week was emotional for several women – session three can often be a turning point when they open up more and begin to really use the group for support. Sometimes, however, some women pull back if they feel they have revealed too much too soon. Timing is such a delicate yet crucial factor. Today's session can also bring up some difficult issues. I wonder what will transpire?

The session

Group process	Comments
Jane (Josh), Helen (Jack), Sonita (Meenu), Jo (Esther), Milka (Janka), Natasha (Simone), Jenny (Lily), Caro (Danny) and Ros (Harry) attend.	
Karen does not attend and there is no message.	
Emma also has not arrived at the beginning of the group.	

Group process	Comments
Check-in	

Jenny begins by thanking the group for their support last week, which helped her get through a difficult week. After the session, she bought herself a large bunch of flowers to cheer herself up and it helped. Jenny was also able to talk to her husband about her feelings, and it turns out that he was also aware of the date but didn't want to say anything for fear of upsetting her. They were able to have an emotional discussion, which was beneficial to them both.

Couples often grieve in different ways and at different rates.

They are also likely to protect each other in this way.

Shared grieving can be mutually supportive.

Natasha was also able to have a heart to heart with her husband. They went out together to celebrate her birthday (their first outing alone since Simone was born) and Natasha was able to tell Martin how excluded she was feeling and how much she missed their previous closeness. Natasha was encouraged to talk to Martin as a result of coming to the group, and now understands the benefits of confronting issues before they become too serious. In her previous marriage, she would bottle up her feelings and then explode, and little would be resolved as her ex-husband would always react with even more anger.

Facilitator observes that both Jenny and Natasha seem to be handing emotional issues in a new and different way.

Sonita is feeling exhausted – Meenu continues to wake three or four times a night, and Sonita has been late getting Asha to school twice in the past week.

Broken sleep and exhaustion are recurrent themes.

Helen and Jane empathise – they too are struggling with broken nights, and they don't have another child to consider.

Helen: 'I know I should sleep in the day when Jack has a nap, but there is so much to do. I used to be so organised, now some days I don't even brush my teeth until 5 p.m., and I don't really know what I do as the house is always in a mess with all the baby paraphernalia. I'm forever washing and ironing and tidying.'

Jenny: 'Ironing? I gave that up a long time ago.'

General light-hearted discussion ensues about short cuts to housework and how chores are divided (or not) between partners.

Helen explains her husband used to do all his own ironing but she feels she should do it as she is at home. 'In some ways I'm looking forward to getting back to work for a rest and I hope it will feel more equal again. I fear I'm turning into my mother, or even my mother-in-law – help!'

Jane: 'Oh, Helen, you shouldn't say that. I don't know what I would do without my mum – she's always on hand if I need her – oh, sorry Caro, I didn't mean to upset you.'

Jane and Helen have very different personalities and attitudes.

Caro assures Jane that she is OK and she's glad Jane's mum is such a support.

Last week Caro disclosed that her mother died three years ago and she still misses her dreadfully.

Group process	Comments
Ros and Jo have discovered they live close to each other, and have seen each other during the week for a walk and a cup of tea. Both comment on the difference this has made, and they plan to meet at the park the following afternoon, weather permitting. They extend an open invitation to anyone who would like to join them.	Alliances and friendships often begin to form during the course of the group.
	The facilitator is just about to bring the check-in to a close when Emma arrives, looking flustered and hot. The facilitator gives her time to settle herself as she makes her a coffee. The group welcomes back Emma, who seems rather surprised by their warmth. She is invited to check-in.
Emma: 'Sorry I couldn't make it last week – Sophie (aged 4) had an ear infection and my two-year-old, Joe, has been really clingy and wants me to cuddle him all the time. He was doing well with his potty training and now he's gone right back, having accidents every five minutes. Anyway, this one's on the bottle now – I can't be doing with breast-feeding all the time. I've kept going as long as I could and she'll go on to solids soon, so it's time for me to stop. She's always had one bottle a day and now she's on it full-time, which is better apart from all the sterilising – I hate that bit.'	As Emma is talking, she starts to make up a bottle for Amy. Amy is fretful and her cries become more urgent. This sets off several of the other babies and the noise level in the room rises, and Emma has to almost shout to be heard. Amy quietens as soon as she starts feeding and Emma starts to relax. The atmosphere gradually calms again as the other babies settle.
A discussion begins on the pros and cons of breast versus bottle, when Jane addresses Emma: 'It's such a shame to give up now Emma when you have done so well and we all know that breast-feeding is so much better for the baby.'	Tension rises again as Emma feels criticised by Jane.
Emma: 'What with my other half being on nights to earn some extra money, trying to keep the kids quiet in the day so he can get some sleep, I'm at my wits end. You're lucky Jane, you have only one child to think about – I have three.'	Emma is on the verge of tears, but is also clearly angry about Jane's comment.
Sonita: 'Actually, Emma, I think you have done the right thing, and I must say I'm thinking of giving up breast-feeding as well. I'm finding it exhausting this time, but I feel so bad about it – all that guilt. And my mum doesn't help. She is forever telling me that none of us ever had a bottle. But I don't feel I can go on with it either – I just want my body back.'	Facilitator maintains a neutral position, while encouraging everyone to express their views on this emotive issue. She emphasises there is *no right way* – whatever feels comfortable for the mother will be the best decision.
Discussion on feeding progresses and Jo tells of her anguish at not being able to breast-feed, even though she desperately wanted to: her guilt and shame when she realised it wasn't working. She had support from her health visitor, but she still feels sad and has had to work hard at not feeling as if she has failed.	

Group process	Comments
As the discussion come to an end, Jane apologises: 'I found breast-feeding so easy. After all the difficulty I had in conceiving, when I, too, felt I had completely failed as a woman, I was so relieved I could do it. I'm sorry. I know I can be a bit evangelical about it.'	Jane seems now to be aware of the effect of her comments to Emma and the group learns the reason why she made it.
Milka tells the group about 'baby tea', a herbal drink given to babies in Slovakia instead of water. 'Janka loves it and she has also become used to drinking from a bottle, which helps when I want to express breast milk. I get supplies from my family. Would any like to try some for their baby?'	Milka's offer is taken up by the group and she promises to bring some next week.
Discussion develops into differing childrearing traditions. Sonita's mother taught her how to massage her first baby to soothe and relax her. There is a suggestion that perhaps she could meet the group and teach them also.	Already the group are making plans to continue meeting up.

Main topic

Memories of holidays, family get-togethers, grandparents, playing with friends and freedom are all freely expressed.	'What comes to mind when you think about your childhood?'
	Positive memories often emerge initially.
Emma: 'All I can remember is trying to keep out of my stepfather's way. He had a foul temper, especially when he'd had a drink, and my brothers and I would hate it when he came back from the pub. Anything could set him off. I always swore I would treat my kids differently, but now I sometimes lose it with them. I know it's not right but I've smacked the older two a couple of times, and then felt awful.'	Emma seems keen to contribute today.
	Facilitator acknowledges this a difficult issue for Emma to talk about.
Caro: 'I know exactly what you mean. My dad had a fiery temper and would lash out. I never really understood why he got so cross, but he used to go mad sometimes. I'm very like him and I'm worried I'll treat my kids the same way. We only really got close when my mum got ill and now he's so different with my boys. But I still don't understand what I did that was so wrong. I get mad sometimes, but I always try to make sure I explain to Tom why I'm angry.'	Caro and Emma were punished because of their parent's moods, rather than because they had been in the wrong. This is confusing for children and increases their insecurity.
	Facilitator reminds group we can break unhealthy cycles, as well as repeat them, and the fact that Emma and Caro are so aware will help them make different choices.
Natasha: 'It was my mum who did all the shouting – my dad was a real softie. I could always get him to stick up for me with mum.'	Facilitator invites others to comment on discipline in their families, ensuring the focus stays on the effect on individuals and does not develop into a discussion about strategies.

Group process	Comments
Milka: 'My dad was great, too, and hardly ever got cross, but when he did, we all knew about it. I was quite scared of his temper, although it was more the threat of it than what he actually did.'	
Natasha: 'I used to think it was great that I could wrap my dad round my little finger, but now I'm on the other end of things. The boys don't see their dad that often but, when they do, he'll get them anything they want – trainers, DVDs, the lot. I want Martin and I to be more united with Simone.'	Natasha has mentioned her ex-husband before. She frequently finds herself in the role of disciplinarian with her sons, while they have fun with their father.
Sonita: 'My dad had a shop that stayed open late in the evenings and also at weekends, so we didn't see much of dad when I was little. When I was a bit older, I started helping out before and after school, and I really liked dad and I working together, but I wish we could have had more fun together.'	Sonita highlights the importance of the relationship with her father.
Helen: 'I don't remember my dad. He left when I was three. Mum worked full-time and we lived with my grandparents. My grandma was lovely. I used to help her with the baking every Saturday, and my grandad had an allotment and he used to grow all our own veg. I used to wonder about my dad, but I could never ask – somehow I just knew I shouldn't, so I still don't know that much about him. Mum moved in with her partner when I was 13, but that's not been easy either. I think I got in the way – he had no children of his own and he wanted Mum to himself. In the end, I spent more time at my grandparents than at home.'	Grandparents can provide stability and continuity at times of change.
Jenny: 'My dad left, too. As soon as I left school at 16, he was off. My mum never got over it – she's still bitter. I didn't see my dad for years but I got back in contact with him when Matthew was born, and we get on OK now. I like his new partner and he is much happier. My mum finds it hard though. She feels I'm letting her down by seeing Dad, but I really missed him and I'd been closer to him than mum, which was why it was so hard for me when he left.'	Discussion on the diversity of family combinations. Divided loyalties present complications in many relationships.
Jane: 'I feel really lucky that I had such a happy childhood, and so did Steve. He was adopted when he was tiny, but has wonderful parents. But since he's become a dad himself, he's begun to wonder more about his background, and now he's thinking he might try to find his real mum. I'm not sure it's a good idea. He could be disappointed and she may not even want to know him.'	Becoming a parent often evokes curiosity about birth for the adopted adult.

Group process	Comments
Ros: 'I used to wish my parents would split up. They argued all the time – still do, in fact. But they both believe you make your bed etc., etc. – that's why I am such a disappointment to them – in this day and age! They're so old fashioned – they call me an unmarried mother. I don't want to marry. I've seen what it's done to them! I want to create a peaceful home for Harry, but I know I need to learn to control my temper and be calmer myself. Because I saw my parents argue all the time, I'm always ready for a fight – and I always want to win. But I don't want Harry to go through any of that, but I'm not sure how to do it.'	Facilitator reminds group that next week the topic is difficult feelings, so this discussion can be continued in more depth then.
Jo: 'I wish I could be more like you. You were really good the other day in the café when we had to wait over half an hour for a sandwich, and the babies both started crying at once. If I'd been on my own I would probably have slunk out without eating even though I'd paid already. But you dealt with it well – assertive without being aggressive.'	Jo's friendship with Ros seems to be giving her more confidence to speak out.
	Ros looks rather embarrassed at Jo's praise.

Feedback

Helen: 'I want my children to be able to say anything to me; to ask me about anything that's on their mind.'	Time is running short, although it feels as if this discussion could continue for some time, so the facilitator asks each participant to say one idea they have to build a positive and happy family life.

Jane: 'My parents always made me feel safe and loved. I hope I can do the same for Josh.'

Jo: 'I want to give Esther the confidence I never had.'

Jenny: 'I hope Matthew and Lily will always look out for each other. I am an only child and was lonely a lot of the time. I hope Matthew and Lily will get on well and stay close when they're grown up.'

Caro: 'Since my mum died, I've learnt it's OK to cry. I want my boys to know that. I've seen my dad cry since mum died, and it's brought us closer together.'

Sonita: 'Having fun as a family; making time at the weekends to go out together.'

Emma: 'To look at them all every night when they are asleep, when they're all clean and angelic looking, and tell myself that I'm doing OK.'

Natasha: 'To treat them all equally.'

Ros: 'I'm still really cross and hurt by Pete leaving me when I was pregnant, and I told him he could never see Harry. But you've made me think today Helen – maybe Harry will need his dad as he gets older, and I'll try to deal with that and not be difficult about it – thanks Helen.'

Group process	Comments
Milka: 'I hope we can bring Janka up to be bilingual. I speak to her in Slovakian and Phil speaks to her in English – I want her to be proud of both cultures.'	Milka speaks passionately about her cultural heritage.
	This exercise has been surprisingly emotional for the group – the facilitator acknowledges this and suggests everyone thinks a bit more about their past and what they can learn from it to create a secure future for their children.
	Reminder of next week's topic – difficult feelings: Group may wish to think about feelings they most struggle with since the birth.

Facilitator's reflections

+ Check-in is getting longer – nearly half an hour this week, but it seemed important to allow that time, especially when the feeding issue became so emotional. It is such a hot topic: do we (as health professionals) increase the guilt by pushing breast-feeding so much? Some people just don't want to or, like Jo can't, we have got to support them, too, so they don't feel they are not giving their baby a good start in life – must talk to my colleagues about this again, about how we can empower women to choose what is right for them.

+ What a lot of emotion today – they were certainly 'storming' today! If the group can tolerate some conflict, it nearly always bonds them closer together. In some groups, it's just too risky, but this group has a number of spirited personalities, and they seemed to cope and benefit from the different views. I hope it encourages the quieter ones like Jo and Jenny to speak out.

+ Jane has rather rigid views. She managed to some extent to upset Emma, Caro and Helen today, and doesn't find it easy to empathise with others. However, I'm glad she was able to apologise to Emma, but also explain the reasons behind her comment. A useful piece of insight for her – I wonder if she realised that before today? So often we take comments at face value whereas, if we can work out what's behind the comment, we can understand each other so much more. We just need to stop ourselves jumping to conclusions and reacting in the immediate, but try to reflect and think a bit.

+ Partners came in for another bashing again – not helping out enough, not getting it right. It can be a rocky time in a relationship – just when they least expect it. Interesting what Helen said about feeling she should be doing more at home now that she's not working – that seems a common reaction. She is trying to reconcile the demands of career and home life, and doesn't want to compromise either.

+ Milka and Sonita are both aware of their cultural backgrounds and want to honour their traditions, and are both sensitive to the tensions that their children may encounter.

+ I wonder what has happened to Karen today? I do hope she comes back, but

I'm not so s   will. Isn't it funny how it always seems to be the ones who
appear the   nfident at the outset who actually are the most wobbly? Not
sure if I shou   ng her again. I don't want to hound her but, on the other hand,
she might just need a little more encouragement to come back. Think I'll sleep
on it and decide tomorrow.

+ Jo is coming out of herself – I think she is finding her feet in this group and her
  friendship with Ros is probably good for both of them. They can learn a lot
  from each other's qualities.

+ Ros seems to be shifting quite a lot. I think she is really beginning to look at
  herself – all her anger towards her parents and Pete is coming out, and allowing
  a softer side to show. Interesting that she has teamed up with Jo, who is probably
  the quietest in the group.

Supporting notes

By this stage, participants are likely to feel more comfortable with each other as
trust has built over the weeks. This session may provoke some sharing of some very
personal and emotional material, and issues discussed at an earlier session may be
revisited.

Having a child inevitably evokes memories of one's own childhood, and this session
encourages the group to think about different aspects of their childhood. Initially,
there may be an emphasis on all the positive aspects, but if the group feels sufficiently
secure other, perhaps more realistic, recollections may emerge. The facilitator needs
to be particularly aware of who is not contributing to this discussion.

The second half of the session focuses on the future and how the couple may build
a firm framework for their children.

Approaches to parenting

Raphael-Leff believes the mother's approach to pregnancy will set the scene for her
approach to parenting, and again describes the three models.[1]

+ **The facilitator** views motherhood as a 'long awaited, deeply gratifying
  experience'. She completely adapts to the baby's needs and believes 'she alone
  has the intuitive capacity to interpret the baby's needs'. In practice, this may
  mean others, including the father, are pushed away as she 'dedicates herself
  fully to deciphering and meeting all her newborn's needs spontaneously and
  immediately'. She will breast-feed on demand, respond to the baby's every
  cry, keep the baby close to her at night and delay weaning. She will deny any
  ambivalent feelings about her idealised baby.

  The facilitator may have difficulty in sharing the parenting role and, indeed, may
  have little time for her partner during this early postnatal period. A resumption of
  the couple's sex life may be delayed, as the mother is consumed by the powerful,
  developing relationship with her child. The father can easily feel surplus to
  requirements, and is denied the opportunity to build early bonds with his baby.

+ **The regulator** has the opposite approach. She wants to return to her 'real'
  life as soon as possible, and expects the baby to fit in around her life and

expectations. She may plan to return to work after a minimum amount of time, and her maternity leave will be used constructively to get the baby into a feeding and sleeping routine. She will introduce other carers to the baby at an early stage, which will enable her to carry on with the rest of her life.

The regulator will not pander to the baby's needs and, if she is sure the baby has been fed, changed and winded, will see no need to pay any attention if he doesn't settle. She can tolerate crying in a way that the facilitator would find impossible.

✦ **The reciprocator** comes between these extremes and views the baby as 'a potentially whole and multifaceted person with whom they can interact'. Mother and baby need time to get to know each other, and the relationship develops taking account of both the needs of the baby and of the rest of the household. The reciprocator has a flexible approach, and attempts to juggle the needs of all concerned, which can at times lead to tension when balance cannot be found.

Changing approaches

Once again these approaches should be viewed as tendencies: few women will demonstrate an absolute approach. Attitudes also change with time, and the group offers an opportunity for exploration and development of style.

In a safe environment, the facilitator mother may be able to disclose more negative feelings towards the baby, and her own need for some separateness and autonomy. Likewise, the regulator may find herself experiencing unexpectedly strong feelings towards her new baby, which may complicate her intended return to work. The reciprocator may find it impossible to always offer an equitable approach with everyone's needs being met – she may have to accept sometimes someone gets a rough deal.

The group can provide an accepting environment for women to explore a development of feelings in these early months of momentous change.

Thinking of the past

New parents may reflect on their own parents' parenting skills and try to understand their circumstances and actions. This may result in deeper bonds being forged, or may underline and consolidate existing disharmony. The absence of family – owing to death, divorce, separation or adoption – may also be acute. Memories of sibling relationships or the lack of siblings may be taken into account when thinking about future family dynamics.

Each partner may have a very different memory of childhood, and may have been raised with different values and traditions. These experiences will influence their thinking and so choices need to be made to arrive at a joint approach to childrearing, taking account of both parents' wishes. For adults with painful recollections of childhood, this period can produce unwelcome and intrusive memories, which can be hard to handle at a time when most couples expect to feel happiest.

Even for adults who can recall a happy childhood, there may be situations and

principles that they want to impart to their children, which may be quite different from their parents. Although by now the facilitator may know a little about the family background of participants, more information is likely to be shared at this session.

As well as being a potentially emotional topic this week, once more a vast quantity of material can be generated. The facilitator needs to manage the time carefully to allow space for reflection about the past, as well as ensuring sufficient time for an exploration of constructive parenting styles for the future.

The progress of life

To put the discussion into context it is useful for the facilitator to consider the progress of life and to bear in mind the influence of family relationships.

Life before birth

'The womb is the child's first world. How he experiences it – as friendly or hostile – does create personality and character predispositions.' Dr Thomas Verney made this statement in his book *The Secret Life of the Unborn Child* 25 years ago.[2] We have all spent up to nine months in this first environment and, inevitably, must be influenced by what happens during this time. By 24 weeks gestation, the baby is always listening, not just to the maternal heartbeat and stomach rumblings, but to voices and music.

Verney cites several studies that demonstrate the importance of the time before birth:

+ of 2000 women studied in Germany, babies born to women who were looking forward to the birth were healthier – emotionally and physically – at birth and beyond than babies of rejecting mothers.
+ the quality of the woman's relationship with the father was of great importance to the developing infant. Does the mother feel happy and secure or ignored and threatened?
+ a woman in a stormy relationship runs a 237% greater risk of bearing a psychologically or physically damaged child than a woman in a secure nurturing relationship.

During pregnancy, most women try to take extra care of themselves – physically and emotionally – to protect the baby. A pregnant woman can often be seen unconsciously stroking her 'bump' to give reassurance to the baby. However, women are not always happy during pregnancy and trauma and distressing life events do occur. The knowledge that undue stress may impact on the growing baby can only add to the woman's already difficult circumstances, and induce increased guilt. Support rather than judgement is required.

Ambivalence towards the pregnancy can make the early months difficult and generate guilt later on, especially if a termination was contemplated.

Family relationships

The baby is born into a family that may consist of a mother with whom he is already familiar, a father whose voice he also knows, and siblings, grandparents and other

extended family members as well. This family provides us with 'our first school for emotional learning: in this intimate cauldron we learn how to feel about ourselves and how others will react to our feelings; how to think about these feelings and what choices we have in reacting; how to read and express hopes and fears.'[3]

Sue Gerhardt describes 'the unfinished baby' and goes on to explain that 'babies are like the raw material for a self'.[4] The newborn is 'incomplete, needing to be programmed by adult humans'. Just as the baby's body grows and develops dramatically, the baby's brain grows at its most rapid rate within the first year and a half. Because the brain of a newborn is so unformed and delicate, these early months can have a great impact on development. The parents become the baby's 'emotional coach', but their ability to fulfil this role will depend both on their own childhood experience and their current emotional stability.

The growing child

As the child develops within the context of the family, he will be strongly influenced by what goes on there. Parents act as role models, teachers, nurturers, disciplinarians – see brainstorming in session two. These early relationships form the blueprint for all future relationships. Children use all their senses to learn and whether, for instance, they hear kind, loving words or harsh, angry words will influence their view of the world. To the growing child, *whatever* occurs in his environment is normal.

According to the theory of transactional analysis, messages received and absorbed by the child at the preverbal stage of development are called 'permissions and injunctions'.[5] Injunctions are negative messages that are often felt rather than heard, but they can have a very powerful effect on behaviour. Each injunction has a corresponding permission.

Typically injunctions begin with 'Don't' and permissions begin with 'It's OK to'. These messages are absorbed from babyhood until about the age of eight, and continue to influence how the adult feels, thinks and behaves. In loving surroundings, with lots of permissions, the child is valued and nurtured, and he will thrive and grow in confidence and self-esteem. But the child who receives mixed, inconsistent or abusive injunctions will feel confused and anxious. In his eyes, the parent cannot be wrong, so the only possible conclusion is that somehow it is his fault – he is to blame. These early messages will contribute to how the growing child feels about himself and will influence his self-esteem.

Life beyond the family

As the child grows, his horizons expand. He attends nursery, primary school and secondary school. Eventually, he leaves home and lives independently of his parents. During this time, his emotional horizons also broaden: he makes friends and spends time with other families. He will come to realise that other families may operate quite differently to his own, and this can be either an informative or sobering experience.

The emerging adult may be able to take a step back from his family and gain some insight to the family dynamics. He may be thankful to be a part of a supportive family, or he may begin to question the values he grew up with. He may rebel, reject

his parents' lifestyle and forge a very different path.

He may come to realise and accept that his parents are not perfect, although this need not detract from their relationship. Or he may not be able to forgive what has happened to him before he was able to protect himself, and so may decide to distance himself from parental contact and influence.

Frequently, however, the messages received in childhood continue to influence and be reinforced in adult life, often outside adult awareness. Becoming a parent may be the first time the adult has been prompted to consider childhood experiences and influences in any depth.

New parents

Women who have had a happy and secure childhood will find it a rewarding and affirming task to look back. They will be able to look to their own mothers as role models and, even if they want to mother differently, they will have the confidence in themselves to make those choices.

But women with an insecure background who received inadequate parenting may worry that they do not know what to do to give their child a better experience than they had. The resulting low self-esteem and poor self-confidence mean the anxious mother will need all possible support. Sadly, her lack of confidence makes it even harder for her to seek out help, and she may isolate herself from available support. For this reason, it is vital that this type of group has an open door policy, where everyone is invited to attend, otherwise a group of women who would really benefit may be missed.

Differing experiences

Each half of the couple brings a past history to the relationship, and each may have had a very different childhood experience. These differences may be obvious: for example, a different ethnic background, culture, faith and socio-economic status. Even a difference in age between the parents can be significant.

However, there are many other differences that are much less obvious but nevertheless need to be addressed. Even families who seemed to be quite similar on the outside may have operated very differently internally.

Variations in family traditions and attitudes can affect all aspects of family life: for example, the approach to birthdays and Christmas, mealtimes and discipline. The use of everyday objects such as televisions and computers may evoke strong differences and feelings between the couple.

This session encourages the mother to think about her past experience and to explore her family culture, and then to evaluate which aspects she would like to continue and which she would like to discard. It would be valuable for her partner to engage in a similar exploration, which could then lead on to a joint discussion about future decisions around how to bring up their family.

Recurring themes
Family constellation

The presence or absence of siblings will always be a significant factor. Alfred Adler placed considerable importance on the make-up of the family, and was particularly interested in the child's position within the family, suggesting attitudes, personality traits and behaviour might be influenced by birth order.[6] Although many factors apart from birth order may affect the child, the position in the family is always relevant to the individual, and forms a significant part of the family history. It is useful to explore how the family constellation might influence the mother's attitudes to parenting her own children.

In *The Importance of Sibling Relationships in Psychoanalysis*, Prophecy Coles reviews some of what has been written about these important relationships.[7] She discusses Melanie Klein's belief in the importance of siblings: they 'promote emotional development and help in the task of distancing the child from its parents', thus contributing to the child's eventual emotional independence and autonomy. Certainly, the experience of having siblings can teach children to share, to negotiate for what they need, and to manage conflict.

Coles quotes Neubauer, who views the birth of a younger sibling as 'creative' in that it helps the older to better manage his aggressive drives. Kris and Ritvo suggest that the choice of marital partner is always influenced by the sibling relationship. In adulthood, we tend to re-create what is familiar, and unresolved siblings rivalries may well influence future personal and work relationships.[8]

The composition of parents' families of origin can also play a part in determining the size of the couple's planned family. An only child may hope to have several children to ensure the companionship that she lacked as a child; an adult from a large family may wish to give an only child the attention she craved. Adults who took on a caretaking role at a young age may even choose not to have children to avoid being overwhelmed by responsibility and demands of a family.

The relationship with siblings is likely to be the longest lasting relationship we encounter, and a positive experience can prepare us for many challenges in adult life. Sibling relationships offer a unique experience that the parent–child relationship can never replicate.

Family breakdown

Following new legislation in the early 1970s, divorce rates in the UK soared from 27 224 in 1961 to 124 556 in 1972, peaking at 180 018 in 1993. Currently, one in every three marriages ends in divorce. However, many couples now do not marry so the total figures for all relationship breakdowns are difficult to gauge.[9]

It is likely that any support group will include women from the traditional nuclear family (married couple with dependent children), but also women from single-parent families, reconstituted or blended families (incorporating stepparents and stepchildren), adoptive families and families with 'vertical extensions' (elderly parents living with adult children).

In the era of the 1970s, when group members are most likely to have been

children, the majority of mothers were not in full-time employment, and so were most likely to retain custody of the children after divorce. Fathers usually played the traditional provider role, which tended to be less 'hands-on' than fathers today. They may even have lost touch with the family as the children grew up: in acrimonious break-ups, the children could have been used as bargaining tools. In these situations, the children may have grown up with a less than positive impression of the role of the father, and harbour feelings of abandonment. Or they may have idealised the absent father and fantasised that he would return and make everything perfect.

Family loyalty and family secrets

Although many women will happily talk about their family background, others may have worked hard to forget a painful past, or feel shame and distress about events that occurred long ago. Family loyalty can provoke powerful emotions and, although most families have at least a few skeletons, family secrets can be corrosive and destructive. To be given a forum to explore such sensitive issues can be very freeing and healing, but may also evoke feelings of guilt and a sense of betrayal to the family 'code'.

At this session, it may be wise to remind the group about the confidentiality contract, and explain the relevance of recapping on the past: the more we understand the past, and the more self-aware we become, the more able we are to influence the future.

Nevertheless, uncomfortable feelings may emerge if individuals reveal previously unexplored aspects of their life, and these uncomfortable feelings must be acknowledged and respected.

Disclosure of abuse

For some women memories of childhood abuse are recovered or evoked around pregnancy and childbirth, and occasionally this is shared within the safe environment of the group. It may be the first time the woman has had the opportunity to talk about this painful issue, or the first time that any interest in her has been shown. It takes enormous courage to disclose such personal information. She will be very sensitive, not only to the facilitator's reaction, but also to the reaction of the rest of the group, and the facilitator has to be able to safely manage the emotions of the whole group.

The woman may benefit from support beyond what the group offers, and the facilitator can provide her with appropriate practical information about local support groups, counselling agencies, and so on. If the disclosure is received in an accepting and non-judgemental atmosphere, the individual is likely to feel empowered by her actions, and it may well provide her with a first step towards recovery and healing.

However, the facilitator also needs to be aware of how the rest of the group reacts. Some may be shaken by this disclosure, or even unwilling to hear such shocking information. Others may be prompted to reveal their own painful past issues. Some may not show any reaction and, although the facilitator can invite them to respond, some individuals may choose not to express how they are feeling.

Group discussions may remind individuals of past experiences that they choose not to share with the group, but that they find disturbing. Individuals may approach

the facilitator at a later time to talk through these issues or to seek additional support: for example, Karen in the case study.

Changing patterns

Each new parent wants to do their best for their child, and there is often a desire to offer a different or better way of life to the next generation to ensure mistakes of the past are not repeated. However, it seems all too easy for history to repeat itself. Anecdotally, there are plenty of stories about children who did not experience a nurturing relationship with a loving parent, and who grow up unable to express or receive love within relationships.

As time goes by, many parents can be horrified to hear themselves using phrases or behaviour they always meant to avoid. The retort of 'because I say so' to the unending 'why' questions of a three-year-old is a fairly bland example that can nevertheless make the long-suffering parent stop and think.

Whatever out history, we all have the freedom to react against, as well as repeat, cycles of behaviour, and new parents can make active choices to provide a healthy and loving environment for their offspring. Positively parenting the next generation can help heal some of the wounds from the mother's own past, enabling her to let go of old hurts and live more creatively herself.

Facilitator as role model

Many of the skills and qualities of the facilitator contribute to a positive parenting style. Novice mothers benefit from care and nurturing themselves as they gain experience and expertise in handling and knowing their babies. The facilitator is able to model these qualities to individuals and they, in turn, can absorb these and then demonstrate them to others in the group and beyond.

The facilitator cares for the women's needs in the following ways:

+ creates a comfortable physical environment, e.g. warm room, comfortable seating, refreshments
+ provides a safe environment to express and share feelings, e.g. ensure no interruptions
+ treats each individual with respect
+ ensures everyone has the opportunity to speak
+ responds without judgement
+ honours conflicting views
+ maintains clear boundaries, e.g. keep confidentiality, be consistent.

All of the above will contribute to each individual's sense of value, and so will help build self-esteem and confidence. Although this may happen in a small way, it may be the first time that anyone has really listened to them, and so be quite a unique experience.

Parenting style will be influenced by the previous experience of being parented.

Each partner's experience may be very different and some dialogue may be required to arrive at a mutually agreed style.

Parenting style will evolve, continuing to develop over time.

References

1 Raphael-Leff J. *Pregnancy: the inside story*. London: Karnac; 1993.

2 Verney T, Kelly J. *The Secret Life of the Unborn Child*. New York: Time Warner Books; 1981.

3 Goleman D. *Emotional Intelligence*. London: Bloomsbury; 1996.

4 Gerhardt S. *Why Love Matters*. Hove: Brunner Routledge; 2004.

5 Stewart I, Joines V. *TA Today*. Nottingham: Lifespace Publishing; 1987.

6 Sweeney TJ. *Adlerian Counselling*. 3rd ed. USA: Accelerated Development; 1989.

7 Coles P. *The Importance of Sibling Relationships in Psychoanalysis*. London: Karnac; 2003.

8 Kris M, Ritvo S. Parents and siblings: their mutual influences. *Psychoanalytic Study of the Child*. 1983; **38**: 311–24.

9 Office for National Statistics. *Living in Britain: results from the 2002 General Household Survey*. London: TSD; 2004.

CHAPTER 9

Session 5: Focus on feelings

The session
Aim
To deepen sharing by discussing feelings.

Objectives
+ To provide a safe environment to share how we feel.
+ To provide support and reassurance that all feelings are understandable.
+ To explore ways of coping with feelings we are not so comfortable with, e.g. anger and anxiety.
+ To share and develop coping strategies.
+ To promote and encourage self-awareness.

Check-in
+ How are you today?
+ Anything left over from last week?
+ Were any of you able to talk to your partners about our discussions on parenting styles?

Main topic
By this stage of the group process, a strong level of trust has usually developed, which makes it possible to explore feelings in an open and non-threatening way. Often participants are able to share a full range of feelings – the less comfortable ones, not just the more acceptable, positive feelings.

Feelings exercise
Introduce this topic by inviting the group to brainstorm all feelings they can think of on to the board.

Distribute the handout on feelings (Appendix 5A). Ask participants to think about the past 24 hours and tick all feelings they can identify. Ask participants to be as honest

with themselves as possible: they will not have to reveal their answers unless they wish to.

Once the handouts have been completed, **the following questions will stimulate discussion**.

Were the past 24 hours fairly typical for you?
+ Were these feelings within the participant's 'normal' range?
+ Was the previous day different in some way?

What sorts of feelings have you have ticked?
+ Were the feelings similar?
+ Were they very diverse?
+ What were your favourite and most difficult feelings?

Roughly how many feelings did you tick?
+ Just a few?
+ Lots?

Has this exercise told you anything about yourself?
+ This exercise is not a 'test' and there are no 'right' answers.
+ It encourages participants to step back from themselves, which promotes greater self-awareness and, therefore, understanding.

Initial responses to this exercise can pave the way into a discussion of less comfortable feelings, e.g. anger, anxiety, frustration, exhaustion and resentment. Facilitator must emphasise the normality of negative, as well as positive feelings.

Difficult feelings exercise (Appendix 5C)
Invite the group to choose a common 'difficult' feeling.
+ What makes me frustrated/anxious, and so on?
+ What makes it worse?
+ How does my body react?
+ What thoughts come into my mind?
+ What other feelings come up?
+ How does my behaviour change?
+ What helps?
+ What else could I do?
+ What would stop me from trying a new way of managing this feeling?

This can lead into a brainstorming session of safe coping strategies, which encourages the group to learn from each other. (Appendix 5D gives an example of a group's responses to this exercise.)

What are the benefits of expressing feelings?
- How were feelings dealt with in your family of origin?
- Has this experience influenced how you cope with feelings as an adult?
- What happens if you bottle up feelings?
- What happens if you express feelings?
- Is there any discrepancy between what you feel on the inside and what you express on the outside?
- How do you manage this discrepancy?

How can you teach children about feelings?
- How did you learn about feelings in your family of origin?
- What would have been helpful for you when you were growing up?
- In what way do you think you will be able to help your children understand and therefore manage their feelings?

What support do you need to do this?
Explore what individuals have found to be helpful in the past. Sharing information and ideas strengthens the bonds already formed within the group. Useful resources include:
- books – facilitator can provide a list of further reading to include topics such as child development, parenting and personal development
- media – magazines, websites, television
- courses on parenting skills, assertiveness, confidence building
- counselling available in the local area for individuals who have personal issues to deal with.

The discussion can progress on to practical ways in which parents can teach children about their emotional world and how to handle this part of themselves. By encouraging individuals to become more emotionally aware themselves, they will be better equipped to act as a role model, and the child will naturally learn by example.

Feedback
Check how members of the group are feeling at the end of today's session, and suggest they might like to take a spare questionnaire home and ask their partner to complete it. This may create opportunities for dialogue.

Give the group the following thoughts to take away.

How aware are you of your feelings? Try to notice them more during the coming week. Can you put some of the coping mechanisms we discussed into practice?

Preparation for ending
- Remind the group that next week is the final session – how do they feel about the group ending and have they any plans to continue to meet after next week?

+ Facilitator will bring some cake to celebrate the ending (check allergies).
+ Suggest to group that they might like to bring cameras next week for photos.
+ Ask the group to think of anything not discussed so far that they would like to share next week.

Equipment checklist
+ Whiteboard/flipchart and pens
+ Baby box (emergency supplies of nappies, wipes)
+ Baby mats
+ Refreshments
+ Tissues
+ Bowl to collect subs

Group case study 5
Facilitator's preparations
It's pouring with rain today – I hope that doesn't put anyone off. I know Sonita, Emma and Jane walk. I met with my supervisor this week and talked through the group process so far. Was able to explore my feelings of envy for Natasha and, once I realised where they came from, I was able to let them go. It's always surprising just how intense past feelings can be when they re-emerge.

Also talked through the need to manage feelings safely within the group, which is sometimes harder when the babies are being very vocal. It can feel quite chaotic when we are talking about emotional issues. Sometimes the women have to speak very loudly to be heard over the noise of the babies crying and fussing.

In the end, I did send Karen a note saying we had missed her last week and hoped she would be able to come this week – we shall see.

The session

Group process	Comments
Jane, Caro (Danny), Jo (Esther), Natasha (Simone), Jenny (Lily), Emma (Amy) and Ros (Harry) attend.	Reduced numbers today.
Helen is ill this week and cannot attend.	
Caro met Karen in the High Street and thought she was planning to come this week. However, Karen does not arrive.	
Sonita sends a message with Natasha that Asha has an ear infection and is off school, so she, too, is absent.	
Jane attends without her son Josh today. Her husband has the day off and she has left them to do some male bonding!	It is interesting that Jane has come without her baby.
Milka does not arrive.	

Group process	Comments

Check-in

Jo asks if she can start the check-in and talks of her struggle with her body image since she was a teenager, how she found the weight gain in pregnancy difficult and is once again trying to get back to a weight with which she is comfortable. 'I was quite plump at 12–13 – puppy fat, I suppose, but I felt horrible. My periods started early as well, which made me feel even more different to everyone else. I felt a huge lump compared to all the others and one girl in particular really had it in for me – lots of sniggering behind my back and sarky comments. Even my best friend joined in – one day she would be all over me and the next day she would blank me. I hated school then.

Facilitator is surprised at Jo's request as Jo had seemed quite uncomfortable at previous check-ins, but was happy to oblige.

'Looking back, I was probably depressed, but then no one thought children could be depressed. I was miserable and didn't feel like eating anyway. I also thought, if I could be more like them, they would like me. I lost loads of weight but guess what, the bullying went on – they still didn't like me.

'I know now that my parents were worried about me. I have only a couple of photos of me then and I looked ghastly, so I'm not surprised, but I just felt they were giving me a hard time as well. It was terrible –

There is a pause as Jo struggles to keep her voice under control.

This is a very long speech for Jo and she looks drained at the end of it. The facilitator thanks her for honesty and bravery in sharing such personal information. There is clear support for Jo from the other women and especially from Ros who is sitting next to Jo.

'Anyway I got over it, but it took a long time and even now I spend far too much time worrying about my weight – I still think people won't like me if I'm fat!

'So becoming pregnant was really risky and I hate being this big now, but this is what I really wanted to say. These last few weeks talking about families and relationships – it's really hit me – the responsibility of being a parent. I don't want Esther to go through what I went through. I want her to feel confident and good about herself – and then I thought well, if I don't feel good about myself, how can I help her feel good about herself? Do you see what I mean?'

Jo: 'I actually feel good about saying it all out loud. For so long all this stuff had been locked inside my head. It's a relief to talk, and it's been easier today in a smaller group, although I was determined to say it.'

Jo's comments about her weight and food trigger an animated discussion on media pressures around image and particularly the pressures on women to be thin and related anxieties and lack of self-esteem when women don't feel they 'fit' this image.

The facilitator acknowledges the risk Jo has taken in sharing her past with the group.

Group process	Comments
	The group is working well today and the facilitator is able to step back from the discussion of this particularly 'hot' topic. Everyone contributes. However, as time is racing on, she brings the group back to the check-in after several minutes, which then continues uneventfully.
Jane: 'I'm feeling really well, but I'm worried about Steve. I think I said last week that he was adopted and it's never caused him a problem. But in the past couple of weeks he's talking about it all the time. All he knows is that his birth mother was very young but, even so, he cannot understand why she gave him up. Becoming a dad himself seems to have opened up a whole can of worms. It all came to a head at the weekend, and he wasn't able to face work on Monday. The doctor has signed him off work this week, which is unheard of. He's really tearful – I don't know how to help him. I'm used to him being the strong one – he was great during the IVF, he kept me going – and now he's crumbling. I think he should talk to his mum, his adopted mum I mean, but he is worried about upsetting her.	Jane is last to check in.
'This morning I really wanted to come here but didn't want to leave him on his own. But I know that looking after Josh will keep him busy – it seems that Josh is the only one who can bring a smile to Steve at the moment. I hate saying this, but I just needed to get out of the house, so here I am!'	The balance in the relationship seems to have changed, which Jane is finding de-stabilising. Facilitator encourages Jane to explore her feelings further and to acknowledge the complexities of the situation. There are no easy answers to Jane and Steve's dilemma, and it is not within the group's remit to find solutions. Offering Jane space to talk through her feelings is valuable and there is an underlying trust that they will be able to work it out.

Main topic

After a tentative start, the group become quite inventive on the range of feelings identified.	The group brainstorm all the feelings they can think of – all responses are recorded on the whiteboard.
The feelings exercise initially generates slight resistance, as babies have to be accommodated, but soon there is a general jollity at some of the feelings: 'I can't remember when I last felt beautiful/lustful/sexy.' 'What does niggardly mean – and maudlin?' 'Zany – I haven't come across that words for years!'	This pen and paper exercise is a new approach to the session, and some of the group seem slightly ill at ease with venturing outside their comfort zone. Caro becomes distracted as Danny grabs her sheet and tries to eat it. Jane offers to take him to enable Caro to complete the exercise. The facilitator invites the group to discuss the exercise.

Group process	Comments
Jenny is surprised at the strength of her feelings. She is having difficulty with her son Matthew, aged 4. He has suddenly become quite aggressive at pre-school, and this week hit out at another child. Now she feels even some of her friends are avoiding her. The feelings she ticked were very diverse: anger with Matthew, but also guilt as she feels she should be spending more time with him; joy at Lily, but also guilt that she finds Lily so wonderful at the moment. This recent development is undermining Jenny's confidence as a mother, and she is again full of self-doubt.	Although reactions to a new sibling are to be expected. it can be challenging and distressing for the mother as she tries to manage such diverse needs without becoming exasperated herself. There will always be new challenges with the first child, whatever their age.
Emma also identifies with Jenny. Her middle child, Joe, wants to be 'babied' and is demanding of Emma's attention whenever she is feeding or changing Amy. 'I don't have time to think much about how I am feeling – most of the time I just think about the next job to do or how I can get more sleep. But actually yesterday was quite a good day. We had some nice times, which I'd probably forgotten about until I did this exercise.'	This exercise can give a balance to the day.
Natasha has ticked mostly fraught and stressed feelings. 'My stepchildren stayed at the weekend. Nick is 15 and was caught smoking at school, and is in big trouble; and Sarah doesn't like her mum's new husband and asked her dad if she could come to live with us! Poor Martin can't handle all these problems. He had a blazing row with Nick, which seemed to go an all weekend, and I end up trying to be the peacemaker and feel exhausted with it all.'	Natasha is feeling pulled in all directions.
Jane: 'My feelings were all extremes. I'm loving being a mum and Josh is an absolute star; and I feel awful saying this but I feel quite resentful with Steve for spoiling it all with all his problems. I wanted it all to be so perfect and it is, but Steve is really unhappy – I just didn't expect this.'	Jane usually puts a very positive spin on things, so being able to express more uncomfortable feelings is new for her. Facilitator comments that many of the group are coping with feelings of ambivalence, and for some these feelings could not have been anticipated.
Ros describes her feelings since the beginning of the pregnancy as an emotional rollercoaster, with more downs than ups. 'Eighteen months ago I could never have anticipated I would be coming to a group like this. I'd never really wanted children, and when I became pregnant I booked in for an abortion. I thought that was the only answer. But then I couldn't go through with it, and suddenly having this baby was the most important thing in the world. I thought Pete and I would be OK and then when he left me, I was devastated. I've been hurt and angry with him for months, and have felt really sorry for myself. I seem to be coming out the other end, thank goodness, and I'm feeling much better.	Brave of Ros to disclose her early negativity to the pregnancy.

Group process	Comments
'I have a beautiful son and I'm going to make a good life with him. I want to meet up with other women who are bringing up their children on their own — there are plenty of us around and, although I like coming to this group, I do feel different to all of you. You're all so settled, even though you all moan about your partners, I sometimes feel envious that I don't have anyone to moan about.	As Ros lets go of her anger towards Pete, space has been created for her to acknowledge the positive aspects of her life and begin to build a future with more optimism.
'But sometimes I'm glad to be free. I might miss the sex and support, but I don't miss the football or the farting or the other revolting habits all men seem to have.'	Ros turns a serious conversation round by introducing a lighter note and the whole group has a laugh.
Jo: 'I ticked empowered. It's a long time since I felt that, if ever. I'm going to take this home and show it to Alex — I wonder what feelings he would admit to. I also ticked greedy and naughty as I had half a tub of Haagan Daas yesterday, which is not so good.'	The mood remains light, but the facilitator notices that Caro has not joined in any of the discussions. Danny has been trying to eat the feelings sheet, and it is now torn and crumpled. 'How did you find that exercise, Caro?'
Caro: 'I hated it. It felt like being back at school. I can't see the point of all this navel gazing. I'm far too tired to think about how I feel and, however you feel, you just have to get on with it, don't you. I still have to feed and change the baby about 20 times a day; entertain Tom, who won't do anything I say; and then there's the endless washing, shopping, cooking, etc, etc. I just don't know how I feel any more.'	Caro looks increasingly flushed and agitated. The facilitator comments: 'You sound really anxious about all the pressures on you.'
'I'm just not coping; I think I'm losing it. This week has been awful. I don't get anything done. I start to do lots of things and nothing ever gets finished — my house is a tip.'	Caro starts laughing and crying at the same time as she tries to make light of her situation.
	The facilitator hands her some tissues. 'It's OK, Caro, we all have days like this. Can you say a bit more?'
'I have this knot in my stomach all the time and then get worked up over stupid things — like this exercise. I felt stupid and didn't want to do it. I don't want to know how bad I feel. What does that say about me? I don't want to be self-aware — I'm too tired. Oh, I'd love a break from myself —.'	When Caro has explored this issue in more depth, the facilitator opens up the discussion: 'How important is it to be aware of our feelings?'
Caro admits Jo's experience of bullying hit a nerve. Her dyslexia wasn't picked up until secondary school and all through primary school she thought she was stupid. 'When I'm asked to do something different or new, it takes me straight back to that time. I guess I still feel angry about the way I was treated. I always felt so useless.'	

Group process	Comments
Natasha: 'I think I am quite a calm person who can usually cope with a lot. But every so often I blow and have a massive reaction to something fairly trivial. So I don't think I'm very good at knowing how I feel. I let things build up too much, and I would find life easier if I confronted issues as they arose.'	The 'pressure cooker' syndrome.
Ros: 'Before I was pregnant, I was quite unaware of my feelings and tried hard not to let them interfere too much. Looking back, I think I was afraid of confronting myself and so suppressed stuff a lot of the time. Since my pregnancy, I don't seem to be able to suppress anything – maybe that's what drove Pete away as I changed so much – suddenly I was emoting all over the place!'	
Jo: 'I know what you mean. I keep everything inside and, when it gets too much, that's when I go for the ice-cream and chocolate. It always comes out with food with me. Again, I don't want Esther to be like me so I have to change now.'	This comment gives insight into how our emotional relationship with food can be unhelpful.
There is a general discussion on how we learn about feelings and the different ways of dealing with feelings: expressing versus suppressing, bottling up versus 'catharting'.	
Jenny: 'Its my body that tells me what's going on. I always get a migraine when I'm stressed. Usually I get a warning but, if I ignore it, I'm in for a full migraine within about four hours. Over the years, I've learnt to take note of what my body is trying to tell me. It's a good early warning system even though it can be very annoying.'	Identifying links between physical health and emotional well-being can provide an 'emotional barometer'.
	The comfortable mood of the group means they can tackle the 'difficult feeling' exercise with ease but also with humour.
	The facilitator asks the group for a feeling they can all identify with, which could be further explored. After some discussion, they come up with frustration. *See* Appendix 5D for the group's responses.
	The facilitator then invites the group to think about how they will help their children to manage their feelings. Talking about feelings and naming them can begin at an early stage, and help to make feelings more understandable for the child.

Group process	Comments
Jenny: 'Matthew can fly into a rage and hit out if he doesn't get his own way. I try to keep calm, but sometimes I end up shouting myself, which doesn't do either of us any good. I think I need to learn to manage my own feelings before I can help Matthew!'	Jenny needs some reassurance that she is doing OK.
	Facilitator brings session to an end and offers spare copies of the handouts to anyone who would like to take one home to have another look at or share with their partner.
	She also reminds the group that next week is the final session. This is met with some dismay. Facilitator asks the group to think about their feelings around ending.

Feedback

Group process	Comments
Natasha: 'I feel I'm just beginning to get into this sort of group. I hadn't realised what it would be like – I came to meet other people but didn't realise there could be such support from each other. I'd really like to keep on meeting.'	
Jenny: 'I agree. I'm going back to work in a couple of months, but I would really like to keep in touch.'	There is general agreement about this and it is agreed the details can be sorted out next week. The facilitator also asks the group how they would like to celebrate the ending at the final session. It is agreed that she will bring a (large) chocolate cake to share with everyone. She also suggests someone might like to bring a camera for a group photo.
Caro: 'Sorry about my outburst earlier. I don't know where all that anger came from. Actually, it felt very good – I'm feeling calmer now. Maybe I'll take another questionnaire home with me and have a closer look at it.'	As the group is about to finish Caro speaks.
Jane; 'I've got things back into perspective, too. Now that I've had a couple of hours away from Josh and Steve, I'm ready to face it all again – I've really missed them. I want to support Steve and, if he wants to try to find his birth mother, I'll do all I can to help. I wonder if I would have said all that if Josh had been here – don't think so. Wouldn't want to hear my moans about his dad, I suppose.'	Final comment from Jane as she rushes out of the room.

Facilitator's reflections

+ We did have a few absent, but I don't think it was the weather. It's good when they leave a message if they cannot make it.
+ Quite an intimate group today, which I'm sure encouraged them all to say a bit more than they would have done if everyone had been present.

✦ I'm amazed at Jo – she was so confident today. She's changed a lot from the quiet little mouse who came on week one.

✦ Natasha has certainly got her hands full – she looked tired today. Having to cope with a new baby and her partner's children and all their worries. Its hard to deal with that range of ages.

✦ Brave of Ros to speak out about feeling different. I've been very conscious when we've talked about partners that Ros may feel excluded, but I thought she dealt with that very well today – it certainly lightened the mood in the room and that was good for everyone today. We've had lots of high emotion in this group and it's good to laugh as well sometimes.

✦ It would be good to talk about difference with the whole group. We can all feel different – Jo and Caro demonstrated that today. So it's not just about obvious difference such as race or colour, but it can also be painful when we feel we are not accepted. Maybe there will be an opportunity to explore that more next week.

✦ I think we may have lost Karen. Having twins brings specific pressures and at the beginning Karen wanted everyone to think she was supermum. I thought she was starting to see it was OK to have off days. But she took a risk telling me about her termination and maybe it didn't feel safe enough for her after that.

✦ Interesting comment from Jane as she left – it's funny how a throwaway comment can be so revealing. She wants it all to be so perfect – she couldn't have anticipated what would come up for Steve at this time, but it's good that she could own her resentment towards Steve – maybe that will help her deal with it.

✦ A few of them picked up spare questionnaires. Wonder how their partners will react?

Phone call from Milka later in the day with apologies for not attending. Very bad night with Janka and overslept, but good news this morning – first tooth has just come through so she is hopeful tonight will be better. She will be there next week.

Supporting notes

This whole session focuses on feelings. We all have them, but sometimes don't know what to do with them. We may feel at their mercy or view them with suspicion. We differ in how we express and communicate feelings, and the traditional British 'stiff upper lip' has done much to ensure feelings are concealed. On the other hand, we regularly hear of instances when feelings have got out of control and violent or criminal acts are perpetrated.

By thinking about feelings in some depth, the group will be encouraged to explore how they each manage their own feelings and how, therefore, they can enable their children to manage theirs. Parents play a huge role in helping the emotional development of their children, which needs to take place alongside their physical and educational development.

The feelings exercise

Brainstorming feelings is a gentle lead into this area and within a few minutes the board is usually covered with a wide variety of feelings.

Asking the group to participate in a written exercise is a new departure and may produce some inhibitions. Some of the women may feel self-conscious, or negative school memories can produce anxiety about 'getting the right answer'. There are also practical difficulties. It is not easy to think, write, hold and feed a baby all at once. But the urgent need to change a nappy or feed an apparently content baby may be a way of avoiding confronting this subject area. The facilitator needs to be aware of this and to reassure individuals where appropriate. As always, participants will be asked to disclose only as much information as they feel comfortable with.

The structure of the discussion this week takes the group through a series of steps that encourages each individual to assess how they deal with their own feelings, and how they have arrived at this method. Some will be very comfortable in both talking and expressing their feelings, while others will be much more reticent or even worried about delving deeper.

Defences developed in childhood may still be in place to protect the individual. However, in adulthood there may be other, more constructive ways of looking after ourselves at an emotional level, and this exercise can prepare the way for this discussion. However, it is important for the facilitator to respect individual defences against articulating emotions. It is equally important to acknowledge and respect emotions (tears, anger, and so on) when they arise in the session.

Shades of feelings

The universal greeting of 'Hi, how are you?' is almost always answered by 'Fine, how are you?'. In these circumstances we are not actually interested in how the other person is really feeling, and would be rather taken aback if we were given detail about what was really happening for the other. Although we might pay lip service to asking, we are not interested in the answer.

At the group check-in, 'I'm fine' is also a way of not saying very much. As the weeks progress, the facilitator can encourage the participants to say a little more about how they actually feel. The feelings exercise can add to the 'feelings vocabulary' of the group, and encourage individuals to be more precise about how they feel. Angry, irritated, furious, annoyed or happy, ecstatic, joyful, content may come from the same family of feelings, yet each has a distinct meaning. Becoming more aware of how we feel can help us deal with feelings.

'Difficult' feelings

The exercise on 'difficult' feelings highlights, and so normalises, the existence of these feelings. There is an expectation that a new baby will bring nothing but warm, cosy feelings and, if other feelings emerge, many new mothers feel guilty and suppress them. If we can acknowledge and identify all our feelings, then it is more possible to find a way through them rather than wasting energy in pretending, even to ourselves, that they are not there.

Fear of anger is common and yet anger is another normal feeling. It is what we do with the anger that can be destructive and make it taboo for some people.

This exercise also encourages the group to recognise the effects of uncomfortable feelings on our bodies and thinking processes. Other feelings may be stimulated, leading to further confusion.

Thinking about feelings in a more integrated way, rather than viewing our emotions as being entirely separate from our bodies and minds, can lead to a more holistic approach to general health and well-being and promote greater self-awareness and understanding of how we each function. This gives us more command of our emotions, promoting stronger self-esteem and confidence.

Difficulties in managing feelings

The family provides the baby with his first experience of relating to others and the 'emotional climate' of the family will colour this experience. A baby from a warm, supportive environment will have a different view of the world to a baby brought up in a family where coldness and aggression reign. Many factors will contribute to the emotional culture of the family.

+ The mother's own ability to deal with her emotions: this will be influenced by her own family background and what she has learnt form her parents, but will also be affected by her current life circumstances.
+ Unacceptability of emotion: in some households any expression of feelings is discouraged or can even be unsafe. This may be related to gender – 'big boys don't cry' and 'nice girls don't get angry' – or it may be that the emotional temperature is so volatile that it is safer to appear quiet and calm whatever else is going on.
+ Depression, especially PND: depression affects the whole family, not just the sufferer.
+ Stresses ranging from physical/external problems (poverty, housing, financial, work-related issues) to emotional/internal problems (bereavement, relationship issues). Ongoing stress with no end in sight can be more damaging than short-term stress.

The number and gravity of the family's worries will also affect how these difficulties impact on the child. If the parents become completely overwhelmed by their own emotions, they will be much less available for their children.

Negative ways of dealing with life stress

+ Suppressing feelings.
+ Withdrawing from the relationship.
+ Isolating oneself.
+ Displacement of feelings – transferring feelings to another arena.
+ Use of artificial stimulants or relaxants – alcohol, drugs.
+ Change to eating patterns – comfort eating or not eating.
+ Self-neglect, abuse or harm.

+ Addictions.
+ Retreat to physical or emotional illness.

Although every family will face challenging and distressing times, how the family deals with difficulties will provide a model for the children in tackling their own future difficulties.

It is also important to acknowledge in the group that we do not always confront issues in the best possible way and that, on reflection, an alternate path may have been more constructive. It can be painful to acknowledge this and every support must be given to women if this realisation occurs. It may be all too easy for an individual to feel discouraged and disempowered as she gains insight in to her own process and behaviour. The facilitator can hold the optimistic view that it is never too late to change and learn more positive ways of managing feelings.

Consequences

The second half of *Why Love Matters* is devoted to an exploration of the consequences of the 'shaky foundations' that might make individuals vulnerable to future emotional disturbances.[1] Gerhardt explores how early experience and a lack of emotional self-regulation may affect:

+ physical illness
+ depression in adulthood
+ reactions to trauma in adulthood
+ a lack of empathy for others.

She also suggests links between early experience and personality disorders.

Goleman also points out the hazards of emotional illiteracy, both for individuals and to society as a whole.[2] Aggression, bullying and the rising rates of depression in adults and children result in further problems, with addictions and eating disorders just two of the consequences to society of emotional illiteracy.

The consequences make uneasy reading and so every attempt must be made to support families at this vulnerable time.

Emotional literacy

Susie Orbach describes emotional literacy as 'the capacity to register our emotional responses to the situations we are in and to acknowledge those to ourselves so that we recognise ways in which they influence our thoughts and our actions'.[3] In other words, 'emotional literacy is the attempt to take responsibility for understanding our emotions'. Orbach explains further the three Rs of emotional literacy:

+ registering an emotional response
+ recognising it – identifying what that response is, which may include giving it a name
+ querying it – is that all of what we feel or is there more to it?

Understanding our own emotions may seem a simple task, but how often have

you been surprised at your response to a particular incident, or how often have you realised that you have ambivalent or even opposing feelings to the same event. Emotional literacy helps answers some of the following questions.

✦ Why do I feel this way?
✦ Why do I do what I do?
✦ Why do I keep finding myself in this situation/relationship/job (etc)?

Emotional intelligence (EI)

In order to be emotionally literate, we need to be emotionally intelligent. Daniel Goleman believes that EI matters more than IQ. He argues that, while IQ measures academic success, it does not predict life success. He believes that IQ contributes only about 20% towards the factors that determine life success, leaving 80% open to other factors. He lists these as the ability:

✦ to motivate oneself and persist in the face of frustration
✦ to be able to control impulse and delay gratification
✦ to regulate one's moods and keep distress from swamping ability to think
✦ to be able to empathise
✦ to maintain hope.

He quotes the explanation by Salovey and Mayer that EI has five domains.

✦ Knowing one's emotions – to be aware of a feeling as it is happening.
✦ Managing emotions – to be able to calm oneself down, work through or cast off distressing emotions. This is not to be confused with 'pulling oneself together', which usually means suppressing emotions, rather than dealing with them.
✦ Motivating oneself – this includes the ability to marshal emotions and to be able to control impulses.
✦ Recognising emotions in others – the development of empathy, the skill of putting oneself on another's shoes.
✦ Handling relationships – managing emotions in others.

As the family 'is the first school of emotional learning', parents can help children enormously, not just by modelling EI but by actively helping a child to manage and understand his emotions. Goleman quotes a study by the University of Washington on the effects of 'emotionally intelligent' parenting. The findings of that study demonstrated that the children benefited in the following ways:

✦ a better relationship with their parents – more affection and less tension
✦ got upset less often, and were more effective at soothing themselves when upset
✦ more relaxed biologically, with lower levels of stress hormones
✦ socially more popular, with fewer behavioural problems
✦ cognitively more able to pay attention and so learnt more effectively.

Developing EI

Goleman assesses several programmes that teach EI, with the following being common components:

+ recognising feelings
+ naming feelings
+ understanding the relationship between feelings, thoughts and actions.

Specific skills are required in order to facilitate this process:
+ the capability to manage emotions – to reduce stress, control impulses, delay gratification
+ to understand feelings – to step back to observe oneself, to realise what is underneath the surface level of emotion
+ good communication skills – being able to listen as well as talk at an emotional level
+ being empathic – the ability to see life from another's perspective, which might be quite different from one's own
+ ability to identify patterns in one's own life
+ skills of assertiveness and problem solving.

The group provides the opportunity to experience many of these skills, and it is to be hoped that the participants will be able to continue developing their own self-awareness and, in turn, be able to help their children recognise, name and understand their feelings.

Preparing the group for ending

At the penultimate week it is important to remind the group of the imminent ending to ensure no one is taken unawares and to ensure any outstanding issues are given some space to be explored.

> How we deal with feelings will be influenced by our family of origin.
> The more we understand about feelings, the more we will be able to manage them.
> Parents can teach their children how to communicate at an emotional level.

References

1 Gerhardt S. *Why Love Matters*. Hove: Brunner Routledge; 2004.
2 Goleman D. *Emotional Intelligence*. London: Bloomsbury; 1996.
3 Orbach S. *Towards Emotional Literacy*. London: Virago Press; 1999.

CHAPTER 10

Session 6: Building self-esteem

The session
Aim
Focus on empowerment of individuals and ending the group.

Objectives
+ To explore self-esteem.
+ To give opportunity to share what individuals have gained from the group.
+ To say goodbye to the group.

Check-in
+ How are you feeling today?
+ Any follow up from last week's discussion on feelings.
+ Any comments from partners?

Main topic
Remind the group that today is the last session and that there will be some time later in the session to talk about feelings around ending. Ask if there are any topics that have not been covered already that the group would like to discuss.

The session today aims to consolidate the work of previous weeks by enabling the group to reflect on what they have learnt about themselves and their new role, and to end the group on a positive note.

The first half of the session focuses on self-esteem and the second half is devoted to an evaluation and celebration of the group, with an opportunity for individuals to talk about their feelings around the group ending.

Focus on self-esteem
The facilitator needs to be mindful that this is the final session and attempt to make it fairly light-hearted and upbeat, and not open up new areas for exploration.

Trust has been built over the weeks and the session can focus on what the women have learnt about themselves and how this can increase their self-esteem.

Initially, the discussion focuses on self-esteem in general terms then develops into a more personal exploration. **The following questions will help the discussion.**

What does the term 'self-esteem' mean for you?
+ What other words come to mind?
+ What is the opposite of self-esteem?

Who provides you with a good role model of self-esteem?
+ Perhaps a well-known person, or a family member or friend?
+ What do they do to show they feel good about themselves?

How do you rate your own self-esteem?
It might be helpful to use a scaling method, e.g. on a scale of 0 to 10, where 10 is the best you could possibly feel about yourself.
+ In the past before you became a mother?
+ Currently since you became a mother?

How do you feel about your role as a mother now compared to when the group began?
+ Can you remember how you felt at the first session?
+ How does that compare with how you feel to-day?

What are the gains in your new role?
+ What are the positives about this new role?
+ What have you learnt about yourself?
+ Have you surprised yourself in any way?

Affirmations are positive statements that can help counteract negative thought patterns and increase self-esteem by promoting a healthier state of mind. Ask individuals to complete the following affirmation:

I feel good about myself because I . . .

Explore how children can be helped to feel good about themselves and what the blocks might be.

The second half of the session focuses on evaluating the group process.
+ What did you expect from the group when you first decided to come?
+ How have you actually found the group?
+ What did you like about it?
+ What didn't you like about it?
+ Is there anything else you would have liked to be included?

And what of the future?
+ How do you feel about the group ending?
+ Do you have any plans to stay in touch?
+ Would you come to this group again with a subsequent baby?
+ Say one thing you will take away into the world from the group?

Final feedback and ending

Summary of the group's journey together and space for the facilitator to also share how she is feeling about the group ending. Ensure there is time for everyone to say their goodbyes.

A group photo can be a lasting memento of the experience.

Distribute the evaluation forms and ask everyone to complete them before they leave.

Equipment checklist

+ Whiteboard/flipchart and pens
+ Baby box (emergency supplies of nappies, wipes)
+ Baby mats
+ Refreshments
+ Tissues
+ Bowl to collect subs

Group case study 6
Facilitator's preparations

Last session today. I often have mixed feelings at the end of a group – there is always a sense of achievement that we have got there, and also a sadness that it has come to an end. Over the weeks I have got to know the women quite well, and it's always fascinating to watch the babies grow and develop. A lot has happened in this group, and some of the women have difficult times ahead, but I think there is plenty of support there for each other – they've laughed as well as cried together, which is also bonding. Oh, someone is struggling to get through the door.

The session

Group process	Comments
Karen attends today, the first time she has been since week three. She is first to arrive and takes the opportunity to explain to the facilitator why she hadn't been for the past few weeks. 'I was hoping to chat to you before everyone gets here. After the last time I was afraid of what might come up and I thought it would be difficult to face everyone, especially Jenny again. Somehow I felt they would all know about my abortion, which I know is ridiculous. I thought they would be able to see through me – oh God, now I sound completely mad. But once I'd missed one week, it was too hard to come the next week. And then I met Jenny, of all people, at the swimming pool. She was really friendly and persuaded me to come along for the last session – and I heard a rumour that there would be cake.'	Karen smiles nervously. Clearly she has been struggling with this issue in recent weeks, and it has taken some courage for her to come along today. Jenny's encouragement has made it possible for Karen to come again without losing face.

Check-in

Group process	Comments
Jane (Josh), Sonita (Meenu), Jo (Esther), Karen (Sam and Beth), Natasha (Simone), Milka (Janka), Jenny (Lily), Caro (Danny) and Ros (Harry) attend.	Facilitator passes on messages.
Helen sent a message to say that she will be late as she has a doctor's appointment.	
Emma also sends her apologies. Sophie, her 4-year-old has just come out in chickenpox so she is housebound. However, she wants to keep in touch with everyone so could someone let her know when and where they are going to meet up on their own next time.	As well as tea and coffee, cake is on offer this week, and a party atmosphere develops as everyone joins in.
Caro speaks first. She can stay for the check-in only as Tom is ill and her husband is at home, but has to leave for work shortly. 'I wanted to come, at least for the first bit, as I wanted to thank you all for listening to me moaning last week. It's very unlike me to let rip like that, but it did me the world of good – maybe I should do it more often! I spoke to Matt at the weekend and he said I should ease up on myself. He offered to go in late this morning as he knows this group has been a lifesaver for me. It was so good to be able to talk about mum – it's been less painful somehow, although I still think about her every day. Thanks to all of you.'	
Karen checks in next. She is glad to be here today and makes little reference to her absence in previous weeks. She comments on how all the babies have grown so much since she last saw them.	Karen seems rather nervous at the check-in and deflects attention away from herself by focusing on the babies.

The comment "A return of Karen's defensive humour! Gradually the others filter in and all are pleased to see her again. It is noticeable that Karen is delighted to be so welcomed." appears in the Comments column aligned with the first entry.

Group process	Comments
Jane's husband has returned to work and plans to do his best to find his birth mother. Jane feels he is not so angry with his birth mother but would still like to find her to try to understand her decision. 'I will try to support him as much as I can. This is something he feels very strongly about, but I can't help wishing it wasn't happening right now.'	Jane is coping better with her husband's emotional state, and is also able to own her feelings about the situation.
Milka is celebrating the arrival of Janka's second tooth, and is planning a visit to Slovakia in a few weeks' time. 'When I first came to England the journey back took 30 hours, but now it is so much easier and cheaper to fly. Phil has got to go on a course for two weeks so I've decided to visit my family. I love living here but every so often I have a severe bout of homesickness. My parents are really excited.'	Living so far away from family can be particularly poignant following childbirth.
Sonita also missed the group last week and is glad there are plans to continue to meet after today. 'Although I met lots of people when I had Asha, this group is different. I feel we can talk about how we really feel, rather than how I think I should be feeling.'	Sonita's comments prompt a general discussion about future meetings, and Natasha offers to host a gathering at the same time next week at her house. There is general agreement and Natasha promises to let Emma know the details.
Jo makes a surprising suggestion. 'When we get together on our own do you think we could still check-in like we do here every week? I've found that so useful – just to have a couple of minutes space to say how I am. I hated it the first few weeks but now I realise how helpful it can be.'	Jo seems keen to re-create and continue the group ethos. The group are receptive to the idea.
Ros: 'Well, I have some interesting news. As you know I've been in touch with Pete over the past couple of weeks, and he very much wants to be a part of Harry's life and to help support us financially. We're still sorting out the details. Anyway, he phoned last night with a real bombshell – he's told his wife about Harry! They've had major ructions, but he says he wants it all out in the open. I haven't had time to think it through yet, but what if Pete wants Harry to go and stay with him – how will I deal with that?'	This news has left Ros in a state of shock, and at present she is unsure how this new situation will develop. Ros has some space to talk through her mixed feelings, but there are no easy answers.
Natasha explains some of her history. She has had to get used to her children spending time with her ex-husband's new partner, and she is also the 'new woman' in the lives of her partner's children. 'We've all had to work at it. It was tough at the beginning but it gets easier. I think Martin's ex and I understand each other a bit better now. We aren't in competition with each any more, although at the beginning we were trying to outdo each other. It was pretty horrible but we're both a bit more grown-up now.'	This is the first time there has been a connection between Ros and Natasha.
Ros appreciates hearing about Natasha's experience, and she hopes she is able to call on Natasha for advice and support if things get difficult.	

Group process	Comments
Jenny checks in last. She is feeling good today. She had a long chat with the health visitor about her son's aggressive behaviour at pre-school and the visitor has suggested some strategies that seem to be working. 'Just in the space of a few days, I feel more in control of things. Matthew can still be difficult, but at least now I feel I have a way of dealing with him. I was starting to be resentful towards him, and I'm sure he picked up on that and it made everything worse. For a while everything he did was wrong, which made Lily seem so perfect. I've got things back into perspective – well, for this week anyway! I hope it lasts.'	Jenny is feeling much less agitated than she was last week.
	Caro nods as if she knows exactly what Jenny is talking about.
	When the check-in is complete, Caro leaves but promises to meet up next week and will bring chocolate!
Main topic	
	After a general discussion about self-esteem, the group is ready to take the discussion on to a more personal level. The atmosphere in the room is relaxed, which facilitates the discussion on what could be a sensitive topic.
Natasha: 'My self-esteem has been pretty shaky over the years, but I think I can say now that I'm doing OK. My confidence has grown since I've had Simone, and actually I think I do a good job with all the kids – well most of the time anyway.'	
Jane describes the high expectations she had placed on herself before she gave birth, even without realising it. 'I thought I must be the perfect mother. I had waited so long for this baby and he might be the only one, so I had no room for mistakes. Gosh, it was exhausting. That first week I was terrified by you all and was so worried that I wasn't making the grade! Then you all started talking about negative things and how hard it was. I could hardly believe my ears – I thought we shouldn't be even thinking those things, never mind actually discussing them! I'm much more relaxed now.'	'Only' children can sometimes become the focus of all the parent's hopes and dreams.
	This leads to a dialogue about perfection and the need to get it right all the time. The discussion is gaining pace when there is a knock on the door and Helen comes in. The facilitator welcomes her and thanks her for her earlier message that she would be late. She asks Helen if she would like to check-in, noticing she seems rather distracted.
Helen: 'Well, yes – no, I'm not sure how I am today. I've just been to the doctor and she has confirmed I'm pregnant.'	Helen trails off and bursts into tears. The rest of the group look rather stunned and are not quite sure what to say. The usual congratulations do not somehow seem appropriate. Tissues are found and Helen is given space to talk.

Group process	Comments
'I think I'm in shock. I'm due to go back to work in two months' time. I don't understand how it happened. I don't believe it – I'm sure we had sex only once and even then I was half asleep – just my luck. How will I cope with two babies under 15 months? Mother-in-law will be delighted – she'd love me to have five or six children. I'd planned two at most, but my body has a mind of its own! I used to be really critical of women who got pregnant accidentally – I used to think how could they do that? And now it's happened to me. Actually, that's quite funny I suppose – it all feels a bit surreal. I need time to get used to this and, oh God, what is John going to say? But hey, let's look on the bright side – the diet can go to pot and I'll start celebrating by having a huge slice of that chocolate cake.'	The words come tumbling out.
	Helen starts laughing and the group join in tentatively. The atmosphere lightens once again as stories of 'accidents' or 'surprises' are revealed.
	Helen receives lots of support and offers of help from the others as she gradually begins to absorb her surprise change in circumstances. The cake is passed around again and the earlier party atmosphere returns.
	The excitement of Helen's news has interrupted the plan for the session and, after some time, the facilitator draws the group back to the subject of self-esteem.
	There is no time to complete the affirmations exercise, but the handouts are distributed and the facilitator suggests everyone could look at them later and maybe even bring them to their gathering next week to continue the discussion.
Ending	
	With about 20 minutes left, the facilitator asks for the group's thoughts on the course. Again Jo takes the lead by being first to contribute.
Jo: 'I've really enjoyed it. It has given me a structure to the week. I didn't know anyone in the area before I came and now I have a whole new circle of friends. I'm going to miss coming.'	
Ros: 'I agree and I've realised that, even though my circumstances are quite different to everyone else's, in fact we all have very similar feelings. Looking back, I'm surprised I came at all, especially as I missed the first week – I think I just felt I had to get out of the house. I nearly didn't come back, but I'm glad I made the effort. I didn't think I would talk about Pete. I thought you'd all judge me for having an affair with a married man, but I really thought he loved me – oh, oh didn't expect to cry. I know I've turned a corner but it's still hard.	It is always comforting to others have similar reactions and feelings.
	As Ros's anger towards Pete has lessened, a space has opened for the pain of the loss of the relationship and tears well up. There is a moment of silence as Ros allows some of her emotions come to the surface.
'Oh, I don't like crying in public; can someone else say something. It is good to let it out isn't it. I can't do this at home – whew. I'm OK now.'	The discussion moves when Ros is feeling calmer.

Group process	Comments

Jane: 'I've been so surprised at how open everyone has been, and it's helped me be more honest about my feelings – as much to myself as to everyone else.'

Milka: 'I was also surprised at how everyone seemed happy to talk about such private matters. I didn't expect that, but it's been very nice and I've learned a lot. At clinic this week I met a new mum who is South African. We got talking and I told her about the group. She is new to the area and doesn't know many people so is really keen to come.'

Facilitator notes her details to ensure she is invited to the next group.

Natasha: 'I came along just to meet other mums as I didn't know anyone else with a baby. I thought it would be all baby talk, and that would have been OK, but it's been really different and I've got much more out of it than I thought. It's really felt like time for me. I'm sorry it has come to an end – these past weeks have flown by. I'd like the group to meet for longer.

Even though this experience was a long time ago, Natasha is speaking about it as if it were yesterday, a painful time etched on her memory.

'It's been so different since I had my eldest 12 years ago. I think I was quite depressed in the early months, but no one knew as I was always bright when anyone else was around. But I can remember going for walks with the pram and crying and not knowing why. It was a real shock to the system, and I felt I was such a bad mother that I wasn't enjoying my baby. If I'd come to a group like this then, I'm sure I would have been fine and realised I was as normal as anyone else. My friends from then are really envious when I tell them about this group. We could all have done with it.'

Sonita: 'I felt I'd forgotten all the baby stuff and I knew I'd need to meet other women with new babies. I feel so much more relaxed now and somehow more complete. Not sure what I mean by that, but I've really liked the way this group has made me think more and question why I do what I do. It's built my confidence and helped me understand my own family more. My mum didn't understand why I needed to come to this group – she thought the family support should be enough, but it's helped me talk to her in a different way, and I think we're closer now.'

Helen: 'Well, I think I'd better get my name down now for a group when this next one comes along. I think I'll need it more than ever – is anyone going to join me?'

Helen's news today and her sharing of her vulnerability has had a definite impact on the group. She seems softer and more approachable, and interacts with the others in a more relaxed way.

Group process	Comments
Karen: 'I'm actually feeling quite envious now as I missed so much. I always want everyone to think I cope really well and like to make everyone laugh. I've always been like that. But I think I've found having these twins the hardest thing I've ever had to do, and I had a severe sense of humour failure. To be honest, I couldn't find anything to smile about for weeks on end and I didn't think anyone would be interested in how I felt. I certainly didn't think I could show just how awful I felt. So it was easier to stay at home. Except of course it wasn't easier – I just got more miserable. Jenny, I'm so glad I met you at the pool last week. I only went because Mike dragged me there. But now I realise it might have helped to come here each week, and I don't have to be the funny girl all the time.'	Karen has been quiet during most of the session today, although it has been clear she has been listening carefully to all that has gone on. The facilitator catches her eye to give her some encouragement, Karen nods and then begins to speak. The group are surprised that Karen lacks confidence beneath the 'jokey' surface, and the discussion develops in to exploring the differences between what we present to the world and how we actually are on the inside.
Jenny: 'This group has helped me realise that it is OK to ask for help. Take the problem with Matt. I was worried he was turning into a little monster, biting and hitting other kids.	Jenny has realised that it can be empowering to seek help, rather than a sign of weakness.
'Before I would have felt so awful about it but wouldn't have wanted anyone to know for fear of being judged. But it actually felt good to ring the health visitor and ask for an appointment with her. In a funny sort of way it made me feel better to sort out the problem by asking for help rather than worrying about it all alone. I've confirmed that I'm going back to work in a few weeks time and that feels good, too. So in some ways I'm glad we are ending today. I feel I've learnt a lot about myself, which I really didn't expect.'	
Sonita agrees with Jenny and hopes the support of the group can continue when they meet up in the future. 'It has been such a relief to know that other people have the same feelings as I do. I feel much less isolated and that's great!'	The facilitator thanks the group for all the positive feedback, but asks for asks for any suggestions which could improve the group.
Jane: 'What about a session for the men? The whole fatherhood thing has really knocked Steve in a way neither of us could have anticipated. He could do with talking through his feelings and hearing how other men cope.'	
Jenny: 'Yes, but would the men talk? Rob would run a mile from talking in public about how he feels. You'd have to have it in the evening and offer free booze – maybe he'd come then.'	Further discussion about the merits of having a session just for fathers or a joint parents session. General agreement that there is no support provided for men.
Natasha: 'I think Martin would come – but I'm not sure I'd want him to. I might not have felt able to say the things I did about him if I'd known he was coming here as well.'	
Jo: 'I showed Alec the feelings questionnaire and got him to do it. I was surprised at what he ticked and we had a good discussion about it. I think he's quite envious of this group, and of all the friendships. I think he'd like to meet some of the other dads.'	This provokes a discussion about possible future social events – maybe a barbecue in the summer.

Group process	Comments

Ros: 'I found the week on parenting styles really interesting and would have liked more time to talk about that. I'm going to need all the help I can get to make things different for Harry.'

Sonita: 'My cousin's wife is just pregnant and I think this group would really help her, but I don't think she would come. They got married last year and, although Rishi was born here, Neena moved to England only after the marriage. She's very shy and lacks confidence in speaking English. They are living with Rishi's parents, who are very traditional, and I'm worried that she is not getting the opportunity to mix with anyone outside the family. I've talked to her about this group, but I know she would be very nervous and would find it very strange to talk about family matters. She would probably feel very disloyal. And yet, she could really do with some support.' Sonita has had mixed reactions when she has spoken to her Asian friends about the group and a discussion follows exploring reasons why women may not attend: lack of confidence in speaking English seemed to be a major factor, together with a reluctance to share personal information.

Ideas to promote the group in future are discussed.

Jenny: 'I'd like to do a follow-up group when Lily is about 18 months – just before the terrible twos when the tantrums kick in. That can be another tricky time – when your angelic little baby becomes a horrible monster. That was a real shock to the system and I floundered a bit then.'

Natasha: 'What about a group for parents of teenagers? That's another big challenge.'

This lead to a discussion about future support and possibilities for ongoing groups.

To finish off the facilitator asks everyone to think of one memory they will take away from the group.

'It gave me somewhere to go every Thursday morning.'

'Someone making me a cup of coffee.'

'Hearing other stories and thinking maybe I'm doing OK.'

'Support from others going through the same stage.'

'Realising my partner isn't so bad after all.'

'Not feeling a freak because I'm not ready to leave him yet.'

'Not feeling a freak because I'm looking forward to getting back to work.' 'Someone else believing I am a good mum.'

'Chocolate cake – I think we needed it every week!'

'I've realised how similar we are on the inside.'

Group process	Comments
Pens are found and everyone willingly completes the forms.	The facilitator shares her feelings about the group: it has been a positive and enjoyable experience for her also and she comments on how she has observed not just the visible physical growth of the babies, which is always a joy, but the emotional growth that has also occurred, which may be less apparent, but no less valuable for that.
	There is time for a group photo of all the mums and babies, which will be forwarded to everyone. There is just one more task to complete: 'Before you all disappear, can I ask you to fill in these evaluation forms –your feedback really helps when we re-apply for funding – thanks.'
	Everyone says their goodbyes – lots of hugs and promises to keep in touch.

Facilitator's reflections

+ That was great, but I am exhausted! All that emotion – I'm feeling pretty drained. Think I'll finish that last piece of cake!

+ Shame Emma missed again, but hope they will include her next time. She's got a lot on and always looks exhausted. Not sure she really got what she needed from the group – she has so little time to think about herself and not much support.

+ Ros has come a long way. She and Natasha seemed to get on well today – they're both older and they seemed to understand each other a bit more today. 'Actually, the age range has been quite wide in this group – I think Emma must be mid-20s, but it worked – doesn't always though. Very young mums can feel quite intimidated by some of the older women, who can seem very well-established.

+ Pity we didn't have time to talk about the self-esteem exercise in more depth, but Helen's news had to take priority – she needed that time to get over the initial shock. We were all shocked. She always seemed so organised, but it was so good she was able to laugh a bit at herself – she endeared herself to everyone. Apparently, she came here straight from the doctor's so she'd only just found out – that's quite a privilege really – to be privy to that sort of news so early on. I hope it all goes well. Wonder what her husband will say. I think she'll be fine, though she may be surprised just how much she needs the group in the coming months.

+ I wonder how the others, especially Jane, felt about Helen's news? It must be difficult for women who struggle so much to become pregnant when they hear

of others who fall pregnant so easily, even when they don't want to.

✦ As usual most of them came to meet other mums – they see it as a social group to begin with. Several of them were quite closed at the beginning, but as the weeks went on they really began to see the value in talking in a more intimate way, and they all relaxed into it. By the end, they were able to use the support of the group.

✦ Their confidence nearly always strengthens, as they 'grow' into their new role. This group was quite tough for some of them as they confronted some of their issues. It's quite a delicate balance – it's not a therapy group, but it does heighten self-awareness. Provided we have taken care to build a safe environment, it works well. Karen was the one I worried about most, but it was positive that she came for the last session. I wasn't expecting her – it took some courage to come today after missing a few weeks She told me her counselling starts in a couple of weeks, and she is looking forward to it. I guess the group has provided that catalyst for her – I hope it goes well. It's interesting how present she was for me, in her absence.

✦ As well as all the intense emotion in the group (I think the tissues were needed every week!), we had lots of laughter, which again helped bond the group. It's another good way of expressing and releasing feelings, and can be very healing.

✦ It's always good to have a mix of first-time mothers alongside women who have children already – that way they learn so much more from each other. It depends who signs up, but I feel it enriches the material.

✦ The end of a group always evokes mixed feelings and they often say they want more sessions. But, on reflection, I think six weeks is about right. It gives time for the group to become established enough for them to be able to continue on their own. A longer group would mean more commitment, which I don't think they are often able to give at this stage. We may find the take-up would be less, especially for women going back to work in the near future. Although it's a bit frustrating when it is clear there are issues and we don't have time to develop them, I hope they take them on board and come back to them at a later date. The aim of the group is to ask the questions to enable the women to find their own answers.

✦ Interesting pointers for the future: a follow-up group at the toddler stage is a good idea, and maybe we will think again about some sessions for dads. Maybe I could find a male colleague who would be interested in running them. Offering a group for parents of teenagers would be really useful as it can be another time of adjustment for families. Often children hit teenage years just as the parents reach midlife issues – a real melting pot of emotion!

✦ So, all in all, it went well. I think I'll see some of them again with the next one, and I hope the sessions on their own will continue to flourish. Now must get the dates sorted for the next group.

Evaluation

I can't believe it's a week since the group ended – time has flown by and I want to make some notes for the evaluation so that I can get it out of the way before the next group begins in a couple of weeks.

The annual funding review is coming up soon, and the evaluation reports are crucial to demonstrate the validity of the work. I find it frustrating that we have to continually justify our existence, and that there is constant pressure to target the service to vulnerable groups and, therefore, exclude many women who appear to be coping. It's ironic that if I was prepared to work only with, for example, women who had been diagnosed with PND, or with teenage mums, funding would be simpler. I strongly believe the work we do is relevant to everyone, but I'm on my soapbox again – concentrate on the evaluation.

Attendance

The attendance rate for this group was 88%, which is about usual. I am always surprised at the efforts women will make to come – five attended every week, which shows strong commitment.

Profile of group

Six first-time Mums, including one set of twins. Only the second set of twins that I can remember. Three second-time mums and two third-time mums.

Work

Six plan to return to work; all part-time, except for Helen who had planned to go back full-time. I wonder what will happen now she is pregnant again?

Feedback forms

Much better system this time. Rather than relying on the questionnaires being returned by post, I asked this group to fill in the forms before they left the last session. I remembered to give one to Caro before she left and posted Emma's, and I have them back now. Last time I had only about a 30% return rate despite a stamped addressed envelope – new mothers are just too busy to catch up with bits of paper.

Emma's makes interesting reading. I didn't really think Emma had fully engaged with the group as she missed a couple of sessions and sometimes had to leave early, but her feedback is really positive – a lifeline! Apparently, she had an invite to attend with her second child but couldn't come owing to lack of childcare, but had heard good reports and so wanted to come this time.

Let's have a closer look at the forms.

Reasons for attending

+ To make friends.
+ To meet other mums.
  (both very common reasons given)
+ The first step to getting out on my own.

What I liked most
+ Making friends.
+ Talking openly.
+ Sharing experiences.
+ Being supported.
+ Everyone was honest about what was going on for them.

What I liked least
+ I sometimes felt guilty as other people were having a really hard time and life is pretty good for me.
+ It was too short – I wanted to meet for longer.
+ No crèche – having to find childcare for my other child was stressful.

What I learnt about
+ Myself.
+ Other people's experiences are similar to mine.
+ There are no rules.
+ I need to be more patient with my husband.
+ It's OK to ask for help.
+ I have some issues I need to look at.

I would have liked to talk more about
+ The birth.
+ Relationships.
+ What to expect next (weaning, potty training).
+ Parenting skills.

I would have liked to talk less about
All blank!

What will you do now the group has ended
+ Keep meeting every week.
+ Keep in touch with everyone.
(same comment by everyone)

General comments
+ I'll be recommending it to friends.
+ So good to know I'm not alone.
+ Relieved that others feel the same as me.
+ My friends from work are envious of this support.

Once again a very positive feedback, which is always good but there are some things to work on.
+ A crèche is becoming a necessity. Apart from the comment above, I know of at least two other women who would have attended if a crèche had been provided.

It is easy to assume second- and third-time mums do not need the group, but this group was a 50–50 split with first-timers. I will have to cost it out – renting another room and employing crèche staff will add to the budget considerably, but it's worth a try. Always a dilemma with limited funding: do we have fewer groups with more facilities, or more groups with less facilities?

✦ Timing the group – Sarah booked in but then didn't come as she had to return to work earlier than planned. She had only moved into the area so missed the last group. Sometimes there is a narrow window between being ready to get out and about and returning to work, so maybe it would have been worthwhile for Sarah even to come for a couple of sessions. Karen had been invited to the previous group but asked to defer to this group, and her twins were six months old by then – by far the oldest in the group. I wonder if that contributed to Karen's feelings of being different – two babies, different stage, thinking she should be sorted – who knows. Again, does it work better if the babies are at the same stage or is it helpful to have an age range?

✦ Will try to do a session for dads as a one-off experiment.

✦ I am conscious that the cultural balance is changing in this locality, and this group highlighted the different challenges that women from ethnic minorities face, as well as the similarities in the emotional reactions to motherhood. My aim is to make the groups available as broadly as possible, but there is a dilemma: to offer culturally sensitive groups or work towards integration across the cultures? More thought needed.

✦ This group was pretty typical, although I know we are still missing some women who would really benefit – something to keep working at.

Postscript – 6 months later

Out of the blue, I've just received a new address card from Caro, with a note to say her husband has got a new job and they are off to the West Country. I was thinking about the group when today coincidentally I bumped into Natasha in the High Street, and had a long chat with her. She greeted me with, 'We're still meeting up,' and went on to tell me all the news from the group.

Helen's pregnancy is progressing and she has about six weeks to go. Jo has just announced she, too, is pregnant but it's still very early days.

Ros is working full-time but comes along to the evening get togethers – they all met up for a Chinese last week to give Caro a good send-off. Sounds as if Caro might have some visitors next summer.

Jenny is also back at work, although off at present as her son, Matthew, broke his leg at his fifth birthday party and hasn't gone back to school yet.

Milka and Jo are also working part-time, although both would like to have another baby.

Sonita went back to work but has recently left and hopes to start childminding soon.

Emma doesn't often make it when they meet up, although last time she said she was pleased as her partner has now got a day job and life has calmed down slightly.

Natasha didn't mention Jane and, when I enquired about her, she looked sad. 'We haven't seen Jane for weeks. I know her husband has been off work for a while with depression, so I guess it's a rough time for her. I feel worried about her though – she didn't come to the meal last week and seems to be isolating herself. I think I'll give her another ring. Isn't it funny, Jane seemed so calm at that first session, yet she's had a difficult time and things are still unsettled for her.' I make a noncommittal comment and ask Natasha how she is.

She and Karen have become good friends. The twins are almost walking and get on well with Simone, who has just mastered crawling. I ask Natasha to pass on my good wishes to the others and we say good-bye.

It was lovely to catch up – so often we don't get to hear what happens to them all. They mostly seem to be doing OK, apart from Jane. It's strange that she has distanced herself from everyone – do hope it works out for her.

Hope to see Helen in a group again soon, and some of the others in future. They'll all be able to take advantage of the new crèche.

As for me, I still enjoy running the groups. Groupwork provides a good balance to my one-to-one counselling work. An exciting development is that I have made contact with the health visitor who works within the Asian community, and we are working together to identify how these groups might be relevant to them. The first step is to carry out some research among the women to ascertain their specific support needs and whether they would prefer to attend their own group or join an existing group. Watch this space.

Another idea has been playing around in my mind recently. I've always fancied writing so maybe I'll write a book about these groups – now that really would be a challenge.

Supporting notes

By the final week the group is often very relaxed and at ease. There can also be an 'end-of-term' feeling and a sense of satisfaction around completion. The goal of attending a weekly group with a small baby cannot be underestimated. It is important to acknowledge and celebrate the group's achievements in some way – some indulgent refreshments are always welcome: cake, biscuits and chocolates go down well.

The last week is also time to consolidate the work of previous weeks, and the aim is always to end on an upbeat note.

Self-esteem

Working on self-esteem, and particularly encouraging the group to recognise individual strengths and achievements as a mother, is an empowering way to end the group.

The level of self-esteem will, of course, vary between individuals, and self-esteem will be affected by both external events and inner resources. It must be emphasised again that these groups are aimed at ordinary women. At this time in their lives they are usually with a partner and happy to be a mother. This in no way discounts issues

and problems which may have arisen with the arrival of a new family member, but overall this is often a happy time.

Even for women who previously had a very poor self-image, motherhood can be a catalyst to challenge that image and begin to build a more positive view of themselves. The facilitator can play a part in validating the new mother and encouraging her to recognise her new skills:

+ her care of the baby
+ the baby's obvious growth and development
+ her commitment to attending the group
+ a willingness to learn new skills
+ a desire to break old patterns can all be highlighted to encourage individuals to see themselves in a new light and can be suggestions to help the women complete the next exercise.

Affirmations exercise

Although this is a light-hearted exercise, it may be the first time some women have actually ever thought of identifying their own good qualities and it can present some with a challenge.

+ 'I can't think of anything.'
+ 'Can't I write the things I *don't* like?'

The traditional British stiff upper lip often provides the greatest obstacle to this exercise: an ingrained fear of 'blowing our own trumpet', or of being boastful, persuades us to keep quiet about our achievements and successes. However, with perseverance and encouragement, and once initial feelings of embarrassment and modesty are overcome, the majority of women write an affirmation. They can help each other with this, and if anyone gets really stuck, ask them to consider what their best friend might say about them.

Ending the group

Although this group is relatively short, it can be a significant support at this very vulnerable time, and relationships that begin during this period can be long-lasting and robust. Women need other women at this time, and a shared vulnerability contributes to the quality and durability of relationships forged.

The regularity of attending a weekly group provides an element of security and routine at a time when life can be unpredictable and unsettled. The cessation of this routine may bring up feelings of anxiety and isolation. The facilitator may have become a figure of stability and consistency for the group – part of her role has been to look after and in some small way to 'mother' and nurture the new mothers, inspiring them to gain confidence in their own abilities.

Coping with change

The focus of the entire course has been on reactions to the changes that a new baby inevitably brings and, although having a baby is mainly a positive change, loss (of the

previous life) is also inevitable. So change and grief are inextricably linked. Ending the group, which may evoke further feelings of loss and grief, is another change that has to be accommodated.

Previous endings

Endings can be experienced in many different ways and a mixture of feelings may be aroused – anxiety, loss, relief, anger, guilt – all to varying degrees. Of course the individual's past experience will colour her present reaction – for example, the woman who felt emotionally abandoned by a mother, who was unable to cope and remained distanced from her children's needs after her husband left the family, may again feel abandoned by the ending of the group. For others, the connection may not be as clear-cut but, nevertheless, they may be surprised by the intensity of feelings that the ending evokes.

An ending exercise or ritual ensures the emotional reactions at the last session can be honoured and provides the group with a constructive experience.

Of course, anticipating an ending can be too painful for some and must be avoided at all costs. Not attending the last session may be a way of avoiding such distress, although this is not always a conscious decision, and often all sorts of other reasons are given. It is always useful for the facilitator to keep an open mind and not to jump to conclusions.

New beginnings

Following the ending of the group, the desire to continue to meet demonstrates a positive outcome. The group aims to provide a supportive and caring experience for each woman who attends and the participants often want to continue contact in some way.

Each group will decide the format and context of future contact, and may or may not include babies and partners. Of course, if the group hasn't gelled very well, contact may not continue. However, even under these circumstances, individuals within the group may maintain friendships.

Ending the group also enables the women to take responsibility for their own future support. The ending itself provides a vote of confidence and becomes an empowering experience, whereas prolonged sessions may reinforce the message that formal support is still needed and could therefore be interpreted as disempowering.

A return to work

It is likely that at least some of the group will be returning to work as the group draws to a close. Some women may be eager to pick up the threads of their old life and be looking forward to returning to work, while others may be wondering how they will manage all the demands likely to be placed on them.

The work environment is not always sympathetic to the demands of motherhood, with no allowance made for the needs of the child. Colleagues may be uninterested in the woman's new role. Women returning to work may find their attitude to work has changed during the maternity leave and it is no longer so important to them. Tensions

can be anticipated as new balances between work and family life evolve.

Women returning to work may have a real need to stay in touch with the group to reinforce and validate the mothering aspect of their life as they integrate all the different roles they play.

Evaluating the group

It is always important to spend time at the final session evaluating the group experience. The following stages can be explored.

+ Beginning the group:
  — reasons for attending
  — feelings before the first session
  — reactions to the early weeks.
+ The group experience:
  — did expectations match the reality of the group?
  — what were the reactions to the style of the group?
  — has any learning taken place?
+ Ending the group:
  — what has been gained from attending the group?
  — has anything changed since the beginning of the group?
  — what does the future hold?

By the end of the six weeks, individuals are often able to give more honest feedback than during initial weeks, and it is a useful opportunity to gain ideas and comments for future planning. All groupwork benefits from continuous appraisal, to ensure a fresh and creative approach.

Epilogue

Shortly after I started writing this book, I received notice that funding for Stepping Stones would not continue. Although the groups had been highly valued by the participants and supported by local health professionals, funding was reviewed annually and always uncertain. I was unsure if alternative funding could be found and, if not, the groups would have to end.

Coincidentally, one of the women attending the current group with her second baby asked me when Stepping Stones started and suggested we have a ten-year celebration. I explained why it may not be possible to continue and she immediately wanted to help fundraise to enable the groups to continue.

Around 30 women, who had all recently attended Stepping Stones, came along on a very snowy February evening to explore ways in which the group's future could be ensured. Within six months over £5000 had been raised mainly by two major events – running stalls and teas at the local village country fair and a spectacular family fun day in August to celebrate Stepping Stones 10th Birthday. Although a core group organised these events, practical help was unstintingly given by many women who had attended over several years.

The core fundraising group went on in 2006 to become Stepping Forward, which then applied for a grant from Action in Rural Sussex to fund other community activities to support families in the local area. As well as continuing to support Stepping Stones, they run mother and baby play sessions and offer training sessions for parents on topics ranging from toddler taming to homeopathy for families. All activities are open to the local community at a nominal cost.

I feel immensely proud to be a part of this process, and have been humbled by the hard work and dedication of the Stepping Forward group. There is variety within the group – some are full-time mums, some work full-time or part-time, some are still in the process of enlarging their families. Many have completed their families and so will not be requiring these services for themselves in the future, but have wanted other women to benefit and share their experience. It seems to me that women are often very generous in their desire to help and support each other, especially at this most wonderful yet vulnerable life stage.

Of course, there has been a parallel process going on: Stepping Stones has now matured into Stepping Forward and Stepping Forward is now an entity in its own right with the ability to make its own decisions. The connection with Stepping Stones continues and the values have been carried forward into a new partnership based on mutual respect and understanding. Ten years ago I could not have foreseen the birth of Stepping Forward and it has been a delight to witness its progress.

We can expect the same process as babies mature into adulthood. The foundation parents provide will influence the growing child and play a part in how they lead their adult lives. However, our children can always surprise us and, as they forge their own path in life, we have to let them go – they have grown up.

Lynn Bertram
May 2008

Testimonials from women who have attended Stepping Stones

'I moved to the area when my son was about five months old. I was keen to meet other new mums, as I was finding the whole parenthood experience quite overwhelming as well as delightful. Every aspect of my life seemed to be turned on its head. People at playgroups were very friendly but you didn't often see the same faces regularly enough. At Stepping Stones I found other parents with babies of similar age. We were quickly able to talk about issues facing us as new parents, and to see that we were generally not alone in the challenges we were facing. There was lots of laughter, as well as a sense of support from the other mums. We have continued to meet regularly as a group after the six-week course ended, so the friendships started at the course have developed even more. We still talk about parenting issues, share tips, go out of an evening every now and then. Stepping Stones has made a real positive difference to my life.'

'I was new to the village when my daughter was born and did not attend Stepping Stones. I felt alone, isolated and very overwhelmed with the major change in my life. After the birth of my son I attended Stepping Stones, where I made some great friends and had a chance to realise that I was not the only one having issues. I still rely on this network of friends and their children to help me through the daily challenge of being a parent.'

'I was apprehensive about being a mum. I have attended two Stepping Stones groups (no plans to attend any more!) and both have brought me security in a wonderful and supportive group of friends, and new-found knowledge on ways to cope with challenging situations. Knowing that there is a like-minded person at the end of the phone is amazingly calming, and I sometimes find myself thinking: "Now what would . . . do in this situation?" It helps! Thank you Stepping Stones and long may you continue.'

'I arrived in the area pregnant with my second child. Stepping Stones was perfectly timed for me. The friends I made through the group have been wonderfully

supportive and, in spite of the size (14+ babies), most of us have remained in contact and see each other regularly. The contrast in the level of support through this group compared to my experience with my first child was dramatic. Stepping Stones is very valuable for new mums. Sharing your experience as a parent is extremely important and helps keep your feet on the ground, knowing that you are going through the same as everyone else! Please help keep Stepping Stones alive.'

'A lifeline when I didn't know anyone in the area, which has resulted in a group of truly great friends whom I know will always be there for me to share the good and bad times when bringing up a family.'

Appendices

The appendices include the prompt questions and handouts for each session. It is not always possible to cover the full range of issues during a session and distribution of the handouts provides the participants with more food for thought, and may help initiate a discussion with partners. The appendices can also be sent to anyone who missed a week.

Appendix 1A: Expectations and reality

Think back to your pregnancy.

Describe what you *thought* it would be like at this stage (the early postnatal months).

What is it *actually* like?

Think about your birth experience.

What about the bonding process with your baby?

How is feeding your baby going?

Appendix 1B: Listening

When I ask you to listen to me and you start giving advice, you have not
done what I asked.

When I ask you to listen to me and you begin to tell me why I shouldn't feel
that, you are trampling on **my** feelings.

When I ask you to listen to me and you feel you have to **do** something to
solve my problem, you have failed me, strange as that may seem.

Listen! All I asked was that you listen, not talk or do – just hear me.

Advice is cheap.

And I can do for myself.

I'm not helpless. Maybe discouraged and faltering, but not helpless.

When you do something for me that I can do and need to do for myself, you
contribute to fear and weakness.

But when you accept as a simple fact that I do feel what I feel, no matter
how irrational, then I can quit trying to convince you and can get about the
business of understanding what's behind this irrational feeling. And when
that's clear, the answers are obvious and I don't need advice.

Irrational feelings make sense when we understand what's behind them.

So, please listen and just hear me.

Author unknown

Appendix 2: Roles of motherhood

What is a mother?

Think of all roles, skills and qualities required to fulfil this role.

In what way is your current role different from your mother's or even grand-mother's role?

What choices have you made about becoming a mother to this child?

What kind of a mother would you like to be?

How can you incorporate this role into the rest of your life?

If you intend to return to work, how do you imagine life will be?

If you are not returning to work, how do imagine life will be?

How will you cope with the emotional as well as physical demands?

What can you do to actively look after yourself?

Appendix 3: Changes in relationships

Which relationship has changed most since the birth of your baby?

In what ways have these relationships changed?

How can these changes be managed?

What changes have you noticed in yourself?

What is important for you now?

Appendix 4: Parenting style

When you think back to your childhood, what comes first to mind?

What was your position/role within the family?

What was your family 'culture'?

What was your partner's experience?

What would be your family motto?

What different styles of parenting have you observed?

Taking your own background into account, how would you like your family unit to function?

Appendix 5A: Focus on feelings

Abandoned	Adamant	Adequate	Affectionate
Agony	Almighty	Ambivalent	Angry
Annoyed	Anxious	Apathetic	Astounded
Awed	Bad	Beautiful	Betrayed
Bitter	Blissful	Bold	Bored
Brave	Burdened	Calm	Capable
Captivated	Challenged	Charmed	Cheated
Cheerful	Childish	Clever	Combative
Competitive	Condemned	Confused	Conspicuous
Contented	Contrite	Cruel	Crushed
Culpable	Deceitful	Defeated	Delighted
Desirous	Despair	Destructive	Determined
Different	Diffident	Diminished	Discontented
Distracted	Distraught	Disturbed	Divided
Dominated	Dubious	Eager	Ecstatic
Electrified	Empty	Enchanted	Energetic
Enervated	Enjoy	Envious	Evil
Exasperated	Excited	Exhausted	Fascinated
Fawning	Fearful	Flustered	Foolish
Frantic	Free	Frightened	Frustrated
Full	Fury	Gay	Glad
Good	Gratified	Greedy	Grief
Groovy	Guilty	Gullible	Happy
Hate	Heavenly	Helpful	Helpless
High	Homesick	Honoured	Horrible
Hurt	Hysterical	Ignored	Immortal
Imposed upon	Impressed	Infatuated	Infuriated
Inspired	Intimidated	Isolated	Jealousy
Joyous	Jumpy	Keen	Kind

Laconic	Lazy	Lecherous	Left out
Licentious	Lonely	Longing	Loving
Low	Lustful	Mad	Maudlin
Mean	Melancholy	Miserable	Mystical
Naughty	Nervous	Nice	Niggardly
Nutty	Obnoxious	Obsessed	Odd
Opposed	Outrage	Overwhelmed	Pain
Panicked	Parsimonious	Peaceful	Persecuted
Petrified	Pity	Pleasant	Pleased
Precarious	Pressured	Pretty	Prim
Prissy	Proud	Quarrelsome	Queer
Rage	Refreshed	Rejected	Relaxed
Relieved	Remorse	Restless	Rewarded
Righteous	Rupture	Sad	Sated
Satisfied	Scared	Sceptical	Screwed up
Servile	Settled	Sexy	Shocked
Silly	Sneaky	Solemn	Sorrowful
Spiteful	Stingy	Strange	Stuffed
Stunned	Stupefied	Stupid	Suffering
Sure	Sympathetic	Talkative	Tempted
Tenacious	Tense	Tentative	Tenuous
Terrible	Terrified	Threatened	Thwarted
Tired	Trapped	Troubled	Ugly
Uneasy	Unsettled	Vehement	Violent
Vital	Vivacious	Vulnerable	Weepy
Wicked	Wonderful	Worried	Zany

Appendix 5B: Feelings exercise

Were the past 24 hours fairly typical for you?

What sorts of feelings have you have ticked on Appendix 5A?

Roughly how many feelings did you tick?

Has this exercise told you anything about yourself?

What are the benefits of expressing feelings?

How can you teach children about feelings?

What support do you need to do this?

Appendix 5C: Difficult feelings exercise

Choose a difficult feeling:

When do I have this feeling?

What makes it worse?

How does my body react?

What thoughts come into my mind?

What other feelings come up?

How does my behaviour change?

What helps?

What else could I do?

What would stop me from trying a new way of managing this feeling?

Appendix 5D: Example of the difficult feelings exercise

Invite the group to choose a feeling they can all relate to. This group chose *frustrated*.

What makes me feel frustrated?
+ Never being able to finish a task.
+ My memory doesn't seem to work at the moment.
+ When I can't comfort Josh – he's colicky at night.
+ My husband complaining how tired he is.
+ Having 3 children crying at once.
+ My parents!
+ My mother-in-law telling me how worried she is about Rob working so hard away from home all week – how lonely he must be and how lucky we are that he is doing so well at his job.

What makes it worse?
+ When I'm having a bad day already.
+ When I'm tired or ill.
+ When there is something extra to do in the day, like coming to clinic.
+ When we are trying to get out for school in the morning.

How does my body react?
+ Tense.
+ Headache.
+ Churning in stomach.
+ Want to sleep.
+ Backache.

What feelings come up?
+ Resentment.
+ Anger.
+ Tearful.
+ Panic.
+ Despair.

What thoughts come into my mind?
+ I can't cope.
+ Will today ever end?
+ I'm a hopeless mother.
+ Why do I have to do all this myself?
+ Where's the chocolate?
+ Tomorrow is a new day.
+ I must calm down.

How does my behaviour change?
+ I shout.
+ I cry.
+ I start rushing around.
+ I stew inside but try to be ultra calm on the outside.
+ I try to slow down.

What helps?
+ Taking the pressure off.
+ Not getting uptight if I'm late – and I'm always late now.
+ Deep breathing.
+ Chocolate – lots of it. I have a secret stash at the back of the fridge.
+ Talking to myself out loud – does that mean I'm going mad?
+ Walking out of the room even just for a few minutes.
+ Putting on some music.
+ The thought of a gin and tonic when they are all asleep.

What else could I do?
+ Let go of some of the expectations I have of myself.
+ Remind myself that this stage will pass.
+ Believe that I am doing a good job.
+ Have some 'me' time to recharge my batteries.
+ Feel I have achieved just one extra thing in a day, e.g. a phone call or email.
+ Ask for help from someone I trust.
+ Find a way to spend time alone with my partner.
+ An early night.
+ Remember to eat during the day.

What would stop me from trying a new way of managing this feeling?
+ Old habits.
+ Too tired to think.
+ Too proud to ask for help.
+ No one around to ask for help.
+ Think I should be able to do it all.

An exercise such as this will throw up a variety responses – from the light-hearted to the more serious. All responses are helpful. Laughter in itself can be therapeutic and is not always a denial of feeling.

Appendix 6: Self-esteem

What does the term self-esteem mean for you?

Who provides you with a good role model of self-esteem?

How do you rate your own self-esteem?

How do you feel about your role as a mother now compared to when the group began?

What are the gains in your new role?

Affirmation

> *I feel good about myself because I . . .*

Index

abuse disclosures 139–40
abuse legacies 29
    see also domestic abuse
Adler, Alfred 138
advertising group sessions 41–2
advice on motherhood 10
Ainsworth, Mary 13–14
Andrews, A 25–6, 101–2
anorexia nervosa 81–2
antenatal care
    care guidelines 19
    choice issues 84–5
    role of healthcare professionals 19–20
antenatal depression 21–2
antidepressants 25
appearances, postnatal changes 122
Argyle, Michael 57
assessment and screening tools 24, 44
'attachment parenting' 14
attachment theory 13–14, 25–6
attendance monitoring 43

babies
    early development 13–17, 26
    first weeks 88
    impact on groupwork sessions 60–1
    impact of maternal PND 25–6
'baby blues' 22
babycare practices
    current perspectives 10–11
    past experiences 11
Biddulph, Steve 10, 14

birth experiences 72, 84–7
    and arriving home 87–8
birth order 138
body image 122
Boston, Mary 13
Bowlby, John 13–14
brain development 15–16
brainstorming techniques 51
breast-feeding 10, 18, 59, 70–1, 99–100,
    128–32
    and drug therapies 25
brothers *see* siblings
bulimia nervosa 81–2

caesarean sections 86
career concerns 103–4
'challenge' techniques 51
child development
    concepts and theories 13–17
        Daniel Stern 15
        Donald Winnicott 14–15
        John Bowlby 13–14
        Sue Gerhardt 15–16
    impact of maternal PND 26
    'life progress' concepts 135–7
    pre-birth experiences 135
    see also neurophysiological development
child health records 20
childhood memories 134–5, 137, 138–40
client information sheets 43–4
cliques 57–8
cognitive behaviour therapy 25

Coles, P 138
communication skills
    barriers to listening 56
    counselling techniques 50–1
    discussion techniques 51–2
community liaison 45
confidentiality 37, 54–5
conflict management 59–60
congruence 49
content of sessions *see* themes and topics
contracts 54–5
CORE (Clinical Outcomes in Routine
    Evaluation) system 44
'core conditions' for growth (Rogers)
    49
cortisol 16
counselling sessions 25
    skills and techniques 50–1
    theoretical background 49–50
    see also postnatal support groups
Coyne, JC *et al.* 27
crèche facilities 40
cultural differences 40, 87
    and parenting styles 124–5, 137

data storage 45
depression *see* antenatal depression;
    postnatal depression (PND)
disclosure issues 54–5, 139–40
divorce 138–9
domestic abuse 83–4
'Dr Spock' 11
drug therapy, antidepressant use 25

early weeks 88
    relationship issues 115
eating disorders 81–2, 122
Edinburgh Postnatal Depression Scale
    (EPDS) 24, 44
emotional intelligence (EI) 156–7
emotional literacy 155–7
emotional outbursts
    and group sessions 59
    see also feelings and emotions
empathy skills 49
employment issues 103–4
ending the group 174–5

evaluating and monitoring group sessions
    43–5, 176
expectations of motherhood 69–88, 182–3
extended family
    impact on infant development 135–6
    relationship changes 117–20
eye contact 50

'the facilitating environment' 15
facilitators
    key roles 30, 47
    limits and boundaries 48
    personal qualities 47
    reflection practices 48
    as role models 56, 140–1
    supervision needs 49
    use of counselling skills 50–1
    use of discussion aids 51–2
facilities
    crèches 40
    rooms and venues 40–1
family breakdown 138–9
family life
    past experiences 137–40
    relationship changes 117
    secrets and loyalties 139
fatherhood 119
    changing roles 18–19, 119, 139
    coping with adjustments 102
    current experiences 10
    see also parenting styles
fathers
    attending postnatal support groups 39
    impact of maternal PND 26–7,
        116–17
    impact of past experiences 137
    previous generations 18–19, 119, 139
    relationship issues 114–17
    responsibilities 116, 139
feedback forms 168, 170–2
feelings and emotions 142–57, 191–7
fees for sessions 36–7
    room rentals 41
Ford, Gina 10
friends, relationship changes 120–1
funding course sessions 36–7, 177–8
    room rentals 41

Garber, J and Dodge, K 26
gender differences, impact of maternal PND 26
Gerhardt, Sue 15–16, 25, 136, 155
Goleman, Daniel 155, 156–7
Gomez, L 13
'the good enough mother' 14, 15
GP roles 19, 25
grandparents, relationship issues 117–19
Greene, JM and Murray, D 21
group dynamics 55–6
    and personality traits 58
group identity 36
group psychotherapy 32
group types and sizes 32–3, 38–9
groupwork
    benefits 29–30
    dynamics involved 55–6
    processes and tasks 53–5, 57–60
    theoretical background 49–50
    see also postnatal support groups

handouts 52
Hay, DF 26
health matters see maternal health; mental health
health records 20
health visitors, healthcare roles 20
healthcare professionals 19–20
home births 84–5

ideas for sessions see themes and topics
The Importance of Sibling Relationships (Coles) 138
intelligence 26
    see also emotional intelligence (EI)
introductions and welcomes 53–4

Klein, Melanie 138
Kris, M and Ritvo, S 138

life progress approaches 135–7
listening skills 184
    barriers 56
Lyons-Ruth, K 23, 27

McCarthy, Dr Michelle 28

market research 33–5
maternal health 18–30
    guidelines 19
    personal experiences 18–19
    role of GP 19
    role of health visitor 20
    role of midwife 20
    see also postnatal depression (PND); stress
Maternity Matters (DoH 2007) 84–5
medications see drug therapy
mental health
    overview of common problems 21–2
    see also postnatal depression (PND); stress
midwife roles 20
mirroring techniques 50
miscarriages 81
mission statements 36
monitoring and evaluating group sessions 43–5
mother–baby bonding
    impact of PND 25–6
    influencing factors 85
    session topic 72–3
mother–daughter relationships 23, 27, 83, 118–19
motherhood experiences
    current perspectives 9–11, 18–19
    impact of past experiences 137
    previous generations 11–13, 19
    session themes
        expectations and reality 69–88
        and parenting styles 123–41
        roles of motherhood 90–104, 185–7
    stages of adjustment 100–2
    see also parenting styles
mothers-in-law 118–19
Murray, L and Andrews, L 25–6, 101–2

natural births 84
neurophysiological development 15–16
NICE (National Institute of Clinical Excellence) guidelines
    on maternal healthcare 19
    on mental health problems 24–5

non-verbal communication techniques 50
'the nursing couple' 15

Oates, Dr Margaret 22, 27
only children 120, 138
open questions 51
Orbach, Susie 155–6
'the ordinary devoted mother' 15

parenting styles 123–41, 189–90
    different approaches 133–4
    influence of own childhoods 134–5
partners 114–17
    impact of maternal PND 26–7, 116–17
    impact of past experiences 137
past emotional problems 29
perfectionism 99
person-centred therapy 49–50
personality traits 58
physical changes, postnatal body changes
    122
planning sessions 32–45
    funding and fees 36–7
    getting started 33–4
    group composition and size 37–40
    initial contacts 53
    monitoring and evaluation 43–5
    promotion and advertising 41–2
    time and dates 38, 55
    venues and facilities 40–1, 53
postnatal care
    care guidelines 19
    role of healthcare professionals
        19–20
postnatal depression (PND) 22–9
    causes 23
    diagnosis 24, 27–8
    impact on babies 25–6
    impact on partners 26–7, 116–17
    in males 116–17
    management and treatments 24–5,
        29–30
    protective factors 23
    risk factors 23
    seeking help 28–9
    symptoms 23
    see also postnatal support groups

postnatal support groups
    aims and philosophy 46
    background theories 49
    benefits and value 29–30
    session management 46–61
        dealing with conflict and emotions
            59–60
        discussion and communication
            techniques 50–2
        establishing aims and values 46
        facilitator roles 30, 47–9
        group processes and dynamics 53–60
        housekeeping tasks 55
        presence of babies 60–1
        tasks and techniques 53–61
    session planning 32–45
        funding and fees 36–7,177–8
        getting started 33–4
        group composition and size 37–40
        initial contacts 53
        monitoring and evaluation 43–5, 176
        promotion and advertising 41–2
        questionnaires 34–5
        time and dates 55
        venues and facilities 40–1, 53
    session themes and programmes 65–176
        course content overview 65
        organisation 66–7
        session-1 'expectations and reality'
            69–88
        session-2 'roles of motherhood'
            90–104
        session-3 'changes in relationships'
            105–22
        session-4 'parenting styles' 123–41
        session-5 'focus on feelings' 142–57
        session-6 'building self-esteem'
            158–74
    support and continuing funding 177–8
    testimonials 179–80
pregnancy experiences 79–84
    and life before birth 135
premature babies 86–7
'primary maternal preoccupation' 14
prompts and cues 50, 51
psycho-educational groups 32
psychological therapies 25

theoretical backgrounds 49–50
see also postnatal support groups
psychosis 22
psychotherapy 25
    group work 32
puerperal psychosis 22

questionnaire use 33–5

Raphael-Leff, Joan 21–2, 82–3, 114, 133–4
reflection 48
relationship issues
    changes since motherhood 105–22, 188
    mother–baby problems 25–6
    mother–daughter problems 23, 27, 83
    with partners 26–7, 114–17
risk factors for PND 23
Robertson, James 13
Rogers, Carl 49
role modelling 56, 140–1
room rentals 41
Royal College of Midwives (RCM) 83–4
Royal College of Obstetricians and
    Gynaecologists 84

Schon, Donald 48
screening and assessment tools 24, 44
Sears, William & Martha 14
The Secret Life of the Unborn Child (Verney)
    135
self-care 93, 102–3
self-esteem 57, 137, 158–74, 198
    affirmation exercises 174
self-identity 121–2
session-1 'expectations and reality' 69–88,
    182–3
    key topic 69–73
    group case studies 74–8
    supporting notes 79–88
session-2 'roles of motherhood' 90–104,
    185–7
    key topic 90–4
    group case studies 94–9
    supporting notes 99–104
session-3 'changes in relationships' 105–22,
    188
    key topic 105–7

group case studies 107–13
    supporting notes 113–22
session-4 'parenting styles' 123–41, 189–90
    key topic 123–6
    group case studies 126–33
    supporting notes 133–41
session-5 'focus on feelings' 142–57, 191–7
    key topic 142–5
    group case studies 145–52
    supporting notes 152–7
session-6 'building self-esteem' 158–74, 198
    key topic 158–60
    group case studies 160–9
session-endings 174–6
sex 115–16
siblings 117, 119–20, 138
sisters *see* siblings
The Social Baby (Murray and Andrews) 25–6
social groups 32–3
socio-economic issues 57–8
Sorensen, Bernice 120
Spock, B 11
Stepping Stones
    background to development 2
    feedback 2–3
Stern, Daniel 15, 30, 82–3, 101, 114
stillbirths 81
storage of records 45
stress
    in infants 16
    negative coping strategies 154–5
suicide 22
summarising techniques 50
supervision 49

talking therapies *see* psychological
    therapies
teenage mothers 39
terminations 81
testimonials 179–80
themes and topics
    'building self-esteem' 158–74
    'expectations and reality' 69–88
    'focus on feelings' 142–57
    'motherhood roles' 90–104
    'parenting styles' 123–41
    'relationship changes' 105–22

time demands 115
transactional analysis 136
'the transitional object 15
Tronick, EZ and Weinberg, MK 26
Tuckman, B 55

unconditional positive regard 49
unplanned pregnancy 80

venues 40–1
verbal prompts and encouragers 50

Verney, Dr Thomas 135

Why Love Matters (Gerhardt) 15–16, 155
Winnicott, Donald 14
    associated concepts 14–15
work colleagues, relationship changes
    121
work issues 103–4
written exercises 52

Yalom, ID 32

Supporting Postnatal Women into Motherhood

DATE DUE